Multiple Choice Questions on *Clinical Chemistry in Diagnosis and Treatment*

Second Edition

S K Bangert MA, MB, BChir

Senior Registrar in Chemical Pathology,
Lewisham Hospital, London
Formerly Registrar in Chemical Pathology,
Westminster Hospital, London

P R Fleming MD, FRCP

Consultant Physician, Westminster Hospital;
Senior Lecturer in Medicine, Charing Cross
and Westminster Medical School, London

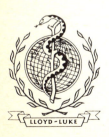

LLOYD-LUKE (MEDICAL BOOKS) Ltd
41 Bedford Square
LONDON

© Lloyd-Luke (Medical Books) Ltd. 1986

First published 1981
by Lloyd-Luke (Medical Books) Ltd.
41 Bedford Square
London WC1B 3DQ

Second edition 1986

British Library Cataloguing in Publication Data

Bangert, S.K.
   Multiple-choice questions on clinical chemistry
   in diagnosis and treatment. — 2nd ed.
   1. Chemistry, Clinical — Problems, exercises, etc.
   I. Title   II. Fleming, P.R.
   616.07'56'076   RB40

   ISBN 0-85324-204-X

Text set in 10 pt IBM Univers
by 🅰️ Tek Art, Croydon, Surrey
Printed in Great Britain by Richard Clay (The Chaucer Press) Ltd, Bungay, Suffolk

Preface to the First Edition

Continuous self-assessment is, or should be, an important part of the learning process. Thus, it is wise, when reading a textbook, to pause from time to time to make a mental resumé of what has been learnt. This collection of multiple choice questions has been published primarily to help those who read *Clinical Chemistry in Diagnosis and Treatment* in their self-assessment. The questions in Part One are arranged according to the chapters in that book and we suggest that after reading a chapter, the corresponding questions are attempted. Reference to the answers will then show clearly the areas in which knowledge is not yet complete and in which immediate revision is required. The questions in Part Two sometimes deal with material from more than one chapter and have been grouped together for those who wish to use them as a 'practice' examination. Most of the questions in this Part are of the *independent true/false* type but some are in the format known as *relationship-analysis*; these are quite searching and, before attempting them, it is important to read the instructions carefully.

Although the questions are all related closely to *Clinical Chemistry in Diagnosis and Treatment* we believe that they will also be of value to those who prefer other textbooks. Whatever the source of information used, these multiple choice questions will be of greatest value if misconceptions and errors of fact revealed by attempting them are corrected immediately.

Dr. J.F. Zilva and Dr. P.R. Pannall have been kind enough to read the questions published in this book and have made many helpful comments. We are very grateful to them for this and for, incidentally, improving our understanding of chemical pathology which is not our own specialty.

P.R.F.
P.H.S.

December 1980

Preface to the Second Edition

We are very grateful to Professor J.F. Zilva for her continuing interest in this book and for her advice on numerous questions. We would also like to thank Dr. Pamela Riches and the staff of the Protein Reference Unit at Westminster Hospital who prepared the protein electrophoretic strip for Question 224.

September 1985

S.K.B.
P.R.F.

Contents

*These questions are arranged to correspond to the chapter numbers of
Clinical Chemistry in Diagnosis and Treatment, Fourth Edition.

Part One

The questions in this part are all of the Independent True/False type; in any question, any number of items, or all or none of them, may be correct.

They are arranged under the chapter numbers of the current edition (4th edition, 1984) of *Clinical Chemistry in Diagnosis and Treatment*.

Chapters I–III
Renal Function, Electrolyte and Water Metabolism

1 Mechanisms concerned in transport across the renal tubular cells include
  (a) passive movement of water out of a tubular fluid which is hypotonic to plasma
  (b) passive movement of anions in exchange for cations actively transported in the opposite direction
  (c) passive reabsorption which continues unchanged however severe an injury inflicted on a cell
  (d) active transport which can be inhibited by ATP
  (e) selective and variable permeability of the tubular cell walls.

2 The following are actively reabsorbed in the proximal renal tubule:
  (a) glucose
  (b) urea
  (c) potassium
  (d) hydrogen ion
  (e) urate.

3 The following statements about countercurrent multiplication in the loops of Henle are correct:
  (a) It probably depends on active transport of ions from the ascending to the descending limb.
  (b) Transport of ions occurs only when the fluid in the loop is stationary.
  (c) Fluid entering the descending limb is almost isosmolal.
  (d) Hypo-osmolal fluid leaves the ascending limb.
  (e) The osmolality of the fluid at the tip of the loop is about twice that of plasma if the urine volume is low.

4 During the production of concentrated urine
  (a) the proximal renal tubules return about 75 per cent of the water entering them to the blood
  (b) the proximal renal tubules present some 40–60 litres of water daily to the loops of Henle
  (c) the osmotic pressure in the renal cortex is higher than that in the medulla
  (d) ADH increases the permeability of the walls of the collecting ducts to water
  (e) the flow of blood in the vasa recta is accelerated.

5 Sodium
   (a) is normally responsible, with its associated anions, for the major share of the osmolality of the glomerular filtrate
   (b) is absorbed in the proximal tubules by passive diffusion down a concentration gradient
   (c) in the distal renal tubule is secreted in exchange for potassium
   (d) when being handled by the distal tubule is influenced by the presence or absence of aldosterone
   (e) competes with potassium in the tubular exchange mechanism for hydrogen ion.

6 Consequences of a reduction in the glomerular filtration rate with normal tubular function include
   (a) oliguria
   (b) reduced urinary excretion of creatinine
   (c) reduced plasma level of urate
   (d) metabolic acidosis
   (e) hyperkalaemia.

7 Renal circulatory insufficiency
   (a) is a recognized complication of mismatched blood transfusion
   (b) is most commonly due to bilateral ureteric obstruction
   (c) does not cause significant ischaemic tubular damage if renal blood flow is restored within a few hours
   (d) is characterized by a high concentration of sodium in the urine
   (e) is typically associated with hypertension.

8 Recognized consequences of predominant renal tubular damage include
   (a) metabolic alkalosis
   (b) hypokalaemia
   (c) polyuria
   (d) inappropriately high urinary sodium concentration
   (e) glycosuria.

9 Recognized causes of renal tubular damage include
   (a) phenacetin
   (b) hypocalcaemia
   (c) hypokalaemia
   (d) Wilson's disease
   (e) galactosaemia.

10 In a patient with generalized renal failure, you would suspect predominant tubular rather than glomerular damage if there were
   (a) a conspicuous rise in plasma creatinine
   (b) urine osmolality approaching that of plasma under conditions of fluid depletion
   (c) a normal or low plasma potassium
   (d) polyuria
   (e) a marked rise in plasma phosphate.

11 In acute oliguric renal failure
    (a) the oliguria is probably due to reduced cortical blood flow
    (b) glomerular function recovers before tubular function
    (c) acidosis in the oliguric phase is later replaced by alkalosis
    (d) urea acts as an osmotic diuretic in the phase of polyuria
    (e) hyperkalaemia persists until renal function has returned to normal.

12 Recognized features of stable and long-standing chronic renal failure include
    (a) polyuria
    (b) a high plasma level of alkaline phosphatase
    (c) hypochromic anaemia
    (d) hypocalcaemia
    (e) normal or slightly raised plasma potassium concentration.

13 The following constitute appropriate therapy for a patient with acute oliguric renal failure due to parenchymal damage:
    (a) high fluid intake to restore urine flow
    (b) intravenous mannitol
    (c) large doses of frusemide
    (d) restriction of sodium intake
    (e) high protein intake.

14 Factors affecting the production of renal calculi include
    (a) a high pH favouring the production of calcium oxalate stones
    (b) residence in the tropics
    (c) inborn errors of amino acid metabolism
    (d) inhibitors of calcium oxalate crystal growth
    (e) a low pH favouring the formation of uric acid stones.

15 The following statements are correct:
    (a) The sodium concentration in sweat is of the same order as that in plasma.
    (b) About half the body water is extravascular and extracellular.
    (c) The normal faecal sodium loss is about 15 per cent of the urinary sodium excretion.
    (d) The total plasma osmolarity is about 500 mmol/litre.
    (e) There is significant sodium loss in expired air.

16 The following ions are predominantly extracellular:
    (a) sodium
    (b) chloride
    (c) magnesium
    (d) phosphate
    (e) potassium.

17 Water
- (a) passes across the cell membrane by a process of active transport
- (b) passes across the cell membrane more rapidly than any solute
- (c) leaves the cells if the extracellular concentration of sodium rises acutely
- (d) moves from interstitial fluid to plasma if the plasma concentration of protein falls
- (e) intake and loss are controlled by the osmotic gradient across membranes of cells in hypothalamic centres.

18 The calculated osmolarity of plasma may not reflect the true osmolality in the presence of
- (a) a plasma urea level of 20 mmol/litre or over
- (b) a serum protein level of 100 g/litre or over
- (c) a plasma calcium level of less than 2 mmol/litre
- (d) gross hyperlipidaemia
- (e) a plasma potassium of 7 mmol/litre or over.

19 Renal sodium retention is favoured by
- (a) a high glomerular filtration rate
- (b) increased secretion of renin
- (c) a decreased secretion of ADH
- (d) expansion of the plasma volume
- (e) a low renal blood flow.

20 Renin
- (a) is secreted by the zona glomerulosa of the adrenal cortex
- (b) is a proteolytic enzyme
- (c) is secreted at an increased rate if the renal blood flow falls
- (d) is in low concentration in the plasma in primary aldosteronism
- (e) is in high concentration in the plasma in secondary aldosteronism.

21 In the assessment of fluid and sodium balance
- (a) total daily fluid loss in sweat and expired air is about 900 ml
- (b) about 500 ml of water is produced daily by metabolism
- (c) daily weighing is a useful means of checking on the accuracy of measurement of fluid intake and output
- (d) it is important to measure the total body sodium
- (e) sodium is important because of the osmotic effect of its concentration in the extracellular fluid.

22 A plasma sodium level of 120 mmol/litre is a recognized consequence of
- (a) prolonged unconsciousness
- (b) Addison's disease
- (c) cardiac failure
- (d) chronic illness
- (e) primary aldosteronism.

23 Consequences of hypovolaemia include
   (a) hypotension
   (b) a fall in haematocrit
   (c) uraemia
   (d) increased urinary sodium excretion
   (e) cardiac failure.

24 Predominant water depletion may be the consequence of
   (a) coma
   (b) nephrogenic diabetes insipidus
   (c) osmotic diuresis
   (d) primary aldosteronism
   (e) prolonged artificial ventilation.

25 Predominant water depletion is a recognized cause of
   (a) suppression of aldosterone secretion
   (b) stimulation of hypothalamic osmo-receptors
   (c) uraemia
   (d) production of urine of low sodium concentration
   (e) low plasma sodium concentration.

26 In a patient who receives a large volume of 'dextrose saline' to
   replace fluid losses from a new ileostomy, the following findings
   would be expected
   (a) hyponatraemia
   (b) passage of small volumes of concentrated urine
   (c) high urinary sodium concentration
   (d) a raised plasma concentration of urea
   (e) a fall in haematocrit reading.

27 In the syndrome of water overloading
   (a) fits can occur
   (b) due to inappropriate ADH secretion, clinical symptoms may
        be absent
   (c) urinary sodium loss decreases
   (d) plasma sodium concentration falls
   (e) oedema can occur.

28 Characteristic findings in primary aldosteronism include
   (a) hypokalaemia
   (b) low plasma bicarbonate
   (c) hypertension
   (d) oedema
   (e) hyponatraemia.

29 Recognized causes of secondary aldosteronism include
   (a) uraemia
   (b) nephrotic syndrome
   (c) cardiac failure
   (d) malignant hypertension
   (e) liver disease.

30 Potassium moves into and/or out of the extracellular compartment by the following routes:
(a) the small intestine
(b) the renal glomeruli
(c) the proximal renal tubules
(d) the distal renal tubules
(e) the walls of all other body cells.

31 Hypokalaemia may result from
(a) prolonged vomiting
(b) constipation
(c) carbenoxolone therapy
(d) diuretic therapy
(e) uncontrolled diabetic ketoacidosis.

32 Factors determining urinary potassium loss include
(a) the ability of the renal tubules to secrete hydrogen ions in exchange for sodium ions
(b) the glomerular filtration rate
(c) the circulating aldosterone level
(d) the amount of sodium reaching the distal tubules
(e) the integrity of the proximal renal tubules.

33 Causes of net loss of potassium from the intracellular fluid include
(a) the administration of glucose with insulin
(b) hypoxia
(c) acidosis
(d) loss of potassium from the extracellular fluid to the exterior
(e) diabetic ketoacidosis.

34 A fall in plasma potassium accompanied by a fall in plasma bicarbonate is characteristic of
(a) renal failure
(b) frusemide therapy
(c) respiratory alkalosis
(d) respiratory acidosis
(e) purgative abuse.

35 Hypokalaemia is a recognized feature of
(a) chronic starvation
(b) renal tubular acidosis
(c) sodium depletion
(d) therapy with acetazolamide
(e) familial periodic paralysis.

36 Clinical causes of hyperkalaemia include
(a) severe injury in a road traffic accident
(b) Conn's syndrome
(c) Addison's disease
(d) severe respiratory failure
(e) renal glomerular failure.

37 Potassium supplementation is desirable for patients being treated with the following diuretics:
   (a) amiloride
   (b) frusemide
   (c) triamterene
   (d) ethacrynic acid
   (e) spironolactone.

38 Consequences of potassium depletion include
   (a) extracellular acidosis
   (b) muscular weakness
   (c) diarrhoea
   (d) cardiac arrhythmias
   (e) renal tubular damage.

39 In the treatment of hyperkalaemia
   (a) frequent determination of plasma potassium simply adds to the patient's distress without improving the standard of management
   (b) intravenous calcium gluconate will lower the plasma potassium concentration rapidly but temporarily
   (c) infusion of bicarbonate promotes movement of potassium into cells
   (d) oral ion exchange resins alone are unsuitable for the emergency treatment of life-threatening hyperkalaemia
   (e) calcium solutions should not be added to solutions containing bicarbonate.

40 Regular measurement of plasma potassium is desirable in patients who are
   (a) aged 75 or over
   (b) receiving oral potassium therapy
   (c) receiving oral diuretic therapy
   (d) receiving treatment with corticosteroids
   (e) being treated for diabetic ketoacidosis.

Chapter IV
Hydrogen Ion Homeostasis

41 Factors which may affect hydrogen ion homeostasis include
   (a) excessive conversion of lactate to pyruvate
   (b) anaerobic energy production
   (c) a high-protein diet
   (d) metabolic release of hydroxyl ions
   (e) violent muscular exercise.

42 The following statements are correct:
   (a) An acid is a substance which can dissociate to produce hydrogen ions.
   (b) A base is a substance which can accept hydroxyl ions.
   (c) Buffering is the process by which a strong acid is replaced by a base.
   (d) pH is the $\log_{10}$ of the hydrogen ion concentration.
   (e) The normal hydrogen ion concentration in extracellular fluid is about 40 nmol/litre.

43 In the measurement of acid-base status
   (a) a decrease of 1 pH unit represents a doubling of the hydrogen ion concentration
   (b) the Henderson – Hasselbalch equation is valid for any buffer pair
   (c) pK' for the bicarbonate buffer system is about 8.1
   (d) it is not possible to measure the carbonic acid concentration in blood directly
   (e) estimation of plasma total CO_2 adequately reflects bicarbonate concentration.

44 Renal mechanisms in the handling of bicarbonate include
   (a) passage through the glomeruli by filtration
   (b) absorption as bicarbonate from the tubular lumen
   (c) dissociation into sodium and bicarbonate ions under the influence of carbonate dehydratase
   (d) diffusion of bicarbonate ion from tubular cells to plasma down a concentration gradient
   (e) active secretion of hydrogen ions from tubular cells into the tubular lumen.

45 Ammonium ion
    (a) forms a buffer pair with phosphate
    (b) diffuses out of tubular cells into the urine much more rapidly
         than ammonia
    (c) dissociates in the tubular cell to liberate hydrogen ions
    (d) produced in the tubular cell leads to increased renal
         excretion of bicarbonate
    (e) is formed from glutamine, together with glutamate which is
         ultimately converted to glucose.

46 Important buffering activity is provided by
    (a) bicarbonate in the blood
    (b) haemoglobin
    (c) phosphate in the blood
    (d) phosphate in the urine
    (e) plasma proteins.

47 'Actual' bicarbonate
    (a) is measured in whole blood rather than in plasma
    (b) estimation normally requires the simultaneous measurement
         of pH
    (c) represents the sum of bicarbonate, carbonic acid and dissolved
         CO_2
    (d) is not significantly different from the plasma TCO_2
    (e) estimation normally requires the simultaneous measurement
         of PCO_2

48 In a metabolic acidosis
    (a) the primary abnormality in the bicarbonate buffer system is
         a rise in $[H_2CO_3]$
    (b) compensation involves a rise in $[HCO_3^-]$
    (c) if compensation is complete the pH is normal
    (d) full correction of all components of the Henderson—
         Hasselbalch equation can only occur if the primary
         abnormality is corrected
    (e) the 'anion gap' is decreased.

49 In calculating the anion gap, 'unmeasured anions' include
    (a) phosphate
    (b) sulphate
    (c) magnesium
    (d) chloride
    (e) urate.

50 The plasma chloride
    (a) in a normal subject accounts for over 80 per cent of the
         extracellular anions
    (b) should be expressed as mEq/litre rather than mmol/litre if
         anion/cation balance is to be calculated
    (c) tends to rise after transplantation of ureters into the colon
    (d) tends to rise in pyloric stenosis
    (e) tends to rise in renal tubular acidosis.

51 In renal glomerular failure
    (a) there is impaired tubular generation of bicarbonate
    (b) there is a compensatory rise in plasma chloride
    (c) the 'anion gap' remains at a normal level
    (d) the plasma pH tends to fall
    (e) respiratory compensation leads to a rise in PCO_2.

52 In lactic acidosis
    (a) there is a compensatory rise in plasma chloride
    (b) tissue hypoxia is a common cause
    (c) treatment with acetazolamide may be responsible
    (d) in the presence of normal lung function the blood PCO_2 is never raised
    (e) an overdose of aspirin may be the cause.

53 Acidosis due to loss of bicarbonate
    (a) may occur when a duodenal fistula is present
    (b) tends to be corrected by renal generation of HCO_3^-
    (c) is unusual unless there is substantial reduction in the GFR
    (d) nearly always requires administration of sodium bicarbonate for adequate correction
    (e) may be due to renal tubular failure.

54 In renal tubular acidosis
    (a) the plasma urea and creatinine levels are nearly always raised
    (b) the tubular cells retain the ability to form ammonia
    (c) urinary phosphate excretion is usually increased
    (d) nephrocalcinosis is a common complication
    (e) the urine pH remains above 5.2 even in the presence of an acid load.

55 In acute respiratory failure causing acidosis
    (a) the arterial PCO_2 is always raised
    (b) the 'actual' bicarbonate may be within the normal range
    (c) hypokalaemia is common
    (d) and complicated by metabolic acidosis, the plasma bicarbonate is always low
    (e) compensation by the erthrocyte mechanism is important.

56 In metabolic alkalosis
    (a) there is marked hypoventilation
    (b) the primary abnormality is a rise in plasma bicarbonate
    (c) tetany may develop in spite of normal total plasma calcium levels
    (d) metabolic compensation depends on increased urinary bicarbonate loss
    (e) with chloride depletion, the urine may be inappropriately acid.

57 Recognized causes of respiratory alkalosis include
 (a) hysteria
 (b) raised intracranial pressure
 (c) chronic bronchitis
 (d) pulmonary collapse
 (e) potassium depletion.

58 In salicylate poisoning
 (a) the respiratory centre is suppressed, causing an acidosis
 (b) the arterial pH is always low
 (c) there may be a metabolic acidosis
 (d) the plasma bicarbonate is usually low
 (e) oxidative phosphorylation may be uncoupled.

59 In a chronic metabolic alkalosis you would expect the
 (a) arterial pH to be raised
 (b) arterial PCO_2 to be lowered
 (c) actual bicarbonate to be raised
 (d) plasma chloride to be high
 (e) plasma potassium to be lowered.

60 Venous blood is preferred for the estimation of
 (a) pH
 (b) PCO_2
 (c) TCO_2
 (d) PO_2
 (e) actual bicarbonate.

61 Measurements on venous blood alone would provide inadequate
 data for the proper assessment of
 (a) diabetic ketoacidosis
 (b) advanced uraemia
 (c) salicylate poisoning
 (d) status asthmaticus
 (e) pyloric stenosis.

Chapters V–VII
Hypothalamus, Pituitary, Adrenal Cortex and Gonads

62 The hypothalamus is the site of synthesis of
    (a) vasopressin
    (b) thyrotrophin-releasing hormone
    (c) ACTH (corticotrophin)
    (d) luteinizing hormone
    (e) oxytocin.

63 In general in endocrine disorders
    (a) negative feedback to a controlling mechanism occurs when the final product of secretion of a hormone falls
    (b) pituitary hormones can be measured with a high degree of precision
    (c) stimulation tests are useful in diagnosis of deficient hormone secretion
    (d) prolonged hypopituitarism may cause the target gland to fail to respond normally to stimulation
    (e) failure of the secretion of a hormone to be suppressed in a suppression test implies normal feedback control.

64 The release of hormones from the anterior pituitary
    (a) involves the passage of impulses from the hypothalamus along the nerve fibres of the pituitary stalk
    (b) occurs intermittently
    (c) is often stimulated by hypoglycaemia.
    (d) may be stimulated or inhibited by hypothalamic hormones.
    (e) in some cases leads to direct effects on peripheral tissues.

65 ACTH (corticotrophin)
    (a) is secreted by basophil cells of the pituitary
    (b) stimulates release of aldosterone from the adrenal cortex
    (c) may cause pigmentation if circulating levels are low
    (d) is secreted in parallel with β-lipotrophin
    (e) deficiency causes Addison's disease.

66 The actions of growth hormone include
    (a) promotion of protein synthesis
    (b) stimulation of amino acid uptake by cells
    (c) promotion of the insulin-mediated uptake of glucose
    (d) stimulation of lipolysis
    (e) stimulation of growth at the onset of puberty.

67 Growth hormone (GH) secretion is stimulated by
    (a) starvation
    (b) the administration of L-dopa
    (c) hyperglycaemia
    (d) exercise
    (e) the onset of deep sleep.

68 In gigantism
    (a) GH excess precedes bony fusion
    (b) there is often accompanying hypogonadism
    (c) death in early adult life is common
    (d) there may be impaired glucose tolerance
    (e) acromegalic features do not develop.

69 In acromegaly
    (a) the increased size of the hands is due entirely to bony overgrowth
    T (b) cardiomegaly is common
    T (c) measurement of basal levels of GH may be inconclusive in confirming the diagnosis
    (d) a glucose tolerance test will depress the GH to less than 10 mU/litre
    (e) development of a toxic goitre is common.

70 Growth hormone deficiency
    (a) can be shown in about half of normally proportioned children of short stature
    T (b) is associated in 50 per cent of cases with deficiency of other hormones
    (c) is not clinically manifest until the age of five
    (d) is diagnosed by measuring plasma GH levels during a glucose tolerance test
    T (e) has a recognized association with emotional deprivation.

71 Recognized causes of hypopituitarism include
    T (a) metastatic carcinoma of the breast
    (b) hepato-lenticular degeneration (Wilson's disease)
    T (c) postpartum infarction
    T (d) acromegaly
    T (e) head injury.

72 In hypopituitarism
    T (a) clinical features of deficiency are usually absent until about 70 per cent of the gland has been destroyed
    (b) TSH is usually the first hormone to be affected
    T (c) aldosterone secretion is normal
    T (d) hyponatraemia is a recognized feature of ACTH deficiency
    T (e) hypoglycaemia during fasting may be a feature.

73 The combined pituitary stimulation test involves the
    administration of
    T (a) insulin
      (b) TSH
    T (c) LH/FSH-RH
      (d) glucagon
      (e) prolactin.

74 In attempting to localize the level of disturbance in a case of
    endocrine deficiency it should be borne in mind that
      (a) a subnormal rise in plasma TSH following TRH injection
          suggests hypothalamic dysfunction
    T (b) a normal, or exaggerated but delayed rise, with TSH levels
          higher at 60 than at 20 minutes, following TRH injection,
          suggests secondary hypothyroidism due to hypothalamic
          dysfunction
    T (c) an isolated hormone deficiency is more likely to be of
          hypothalamic than of pituitary origin
    T (d) in hypogonadism, low basal gonadotrophin levels with a
          delayed but quantitatively normal response to LH/FSH-RH
          suggests a hypothalamic cause
      (e) a subnormal cortisol response to insulin-induced
          hypoglycaemia is unequivocal evidence of a pituitary cause.

75 The following are hypothalamic hormones which are commonly
    available for stimulation tests:
    T (a) thyrotrophin-releasing hormone
      (b) neurophysin
      (c) corticotrophin-releasing factor
    T (d) FSH/LH releasing hormone
      (e) somatomedin.

76 Adrenal androgens
      (a) are synthesized in the zona glomerulosa of the adrenal cortex
      (b) are secreted in excessive amounts in the presence of C_{21}- or
          C_{11}-hydroxylase deficiency
      (c) stimulate protein synthesis
      (d) at physiological levels have little androgenic effect
      (e) are secreted in increased amounts in response to a rise in
          ACTH secretion.

77 Physiological functions of glucocorticoids include
    T (a) stimulation of gluconeogenesis
      (b) control of Na^+/K^+ exchanges across cell membranes
    T (c) maintenance of blood pressure
    T (d) maintenance of extracellular fluid volume
    T (e) a role in the synthesis of adrenaline (epinephrine).

78 In the laboratory investigation of adrenocortical function
T (a) abnormalities of the plasma proteins may cause misinterpretation of results
T (b) estimation of plasma ACTH is helpful in elucidating the cause of Cushing's syndrome
  (c) synthetic CRF is given intravenously in stimulation tests
  (d) measurement of 17-oxosteroids and 17-oxogenic steroids is a reliable test of hormone secretion but is too time-consuming for routine use
  (e) plasma ACTH is usually raised in the presence of an adenoma of the adrenal cortex.

79 Characteristic clinical features of Cushing's syndrome include
T (a) menstrual irregularities in women
  (b) increased muscular strength
T (c) hirsutism
T (d) osteoporosis
T (e) hypertension.

80 Recognized biochemical abnormalities in Cushing's syndrome include
used (a) hypoglycaemia
T (b) hypokalaemia
T (c) accelerated protein breakdown
  (d) hyponatraemia
T (e) water retention.

81 In the investigation of a suspected case of Cushing's syndrome
T (a) loss of the circadian variation of plasma cortisol should be sought as an early sign
T (b) if both plasma and urinary levels of cortisol are normal, Cushing's syndrome is unlikely
T (c) the clinical and biochemical features of Cushing's syndrome can be mimicked by severe alcohol abuse
  (d) in simple obesity, because of a prolonged biochemical half-life of cortisol, plasma levels may be elevated
T (e) endogenous depression may cause marked elevation of plasma cortisol.

82 In Cushing's syndrome
  (a) the short dexamethasone suppression test is valuable in distinguishing between pituitary-dependent adrenal hyperplasia and adrenal adenoma
  (b) failure of the short dexamethasone test to suppress plasma cortisol levels is diagnostic
used
used (T (c) very high plasma cortisol levels suggest adrenocortical carcinoma or ectopic ACTH secretion
  (d) the high-dose dexamethasone test will cause a lowering of plasma cortisol levels in all cases except those due to ectopic ACTH
  (e) plasma ACTH is usually very high in adrenocortical carcinoma.

83 In Addison's disease
   T (a) a normal plasma sodium level is compatible with substantial
            sodium depletion
       (b) estimation of urinary sodium is a valuable diagnostic test
Used (T (c) the glomerular filtration rate is reduced
   T (d) hypoglycaemia is a recognized feature
       (e) failure of adrenal androgen secretion causes impotence.

84 In the investigation of a case of acute adrenal failure
       (a) it is essential to establish the diagnosis by measurement of
            plasma cortisol before starting treatment
   T (b) Synacthen is more satisfactory than ACTH in stimulation
            tests
       (c) the short Synacthen test effectively distinguishes between   a NO
            Addison's disease and ACTH deficiency
       (d) estimation of urinary steroid excretion is valuable in
            distinguishing between primary and secondary adrenal
            insufficiency
   T (e) in suspected ACTH deficiency a full pituitary function test
            should be done.

85 Recognized consequences of C_{21}-hydroxylase deficiency include
       (a) male pseudohermaphroditism
   T (b) female pseudohermaphroditism
   T (c) precocious puberty in the male
   T (d) virilization in the female at puberty   NO
       (e) gynaecomastia.

86 Expected laboratory findings in C_{21}-hydroxylase deficiency include
       (a) low or undetectable levels of plasma 17-hydroxyprogesterone
   T (b) increased urinary excretion of pregnanetriol
   T (c) increased plasma androstenedione concentration
   T (d) raised levels of plasma ACTH
       (e) an abnormally high proportion of 11-hydroxylated steroids
            in the urine.

87 Control of gonadal function in the female involves the following
    mechanisms:
   T (a) A rapid increase in oestrogen secretion stimulates production
            of luteinizing hormone.
   T (b) Progesterone is secreted by the corpus luteum.
   T (c) Sustained high levels of oestrogens and progesterone inhibit
            pituitary gonadotrophin secretion.
       (d) Inhibin reduces FSH secretion.
   T (e) The same hypothalamic factor influences pituitary secretion
            of both follicle-stimulating and luteinizing hormones.

88 During the menstrual cycle,
T (a) at the beginning of the follicular phase ovarian hormone
        levels are low
T (b) rising levels of oestrogen in the follicular phase cause
        regeneration of endometrium
  (c) luteinizing hormone secretion reaches a peak two or three
        days after the onset of the luteal phase
  (d) the corpus luteum secretes progesterone but no oestrogen
T (e) menstrual bleeding is precipitated by falling levels of ovarian
        hormones.

89 Prolactin
  (a) is secreted by the pituitary in response to the secretion of a
        hypothalamic releasing factor
T (b) may be secreted in excess by some pituitary tumours
T (c) is secreted in larger amounts during sleep
T (d) is secreted in increased amounts following the injection of
        thyrotrophin-releasing hormone
  (e) is secreted in increased amounts in nearly all cases of
        gynaecomastia.

90 Raised levels of plasma prolactin may be the result of
T (a) stress
T (b) hypothyroidism
  (c) Sheehan's syndrome
T (d) the use of oral contraceptives
T (e) chronic renal failure.

91 In the investigation of secondary amenorrhoea it is important to
    consider the possibility of
  (a) chromosomal abnormalities
T (b) pregnancy
T (c) hyperprolactinaemia
T (d) gonadotrophin deficiency
  (e) delayed puberty.

92 Recognized causes of virilism in the female include
T (a) ovarian arrhenoblastoma
  (b) polycystic ovaries
T (c) congenital adrenal hyperplasia
  (d) a familial predisposition
T (e) pituitary-dependent Cushing's syndrome.

93 Clomiphene
   T (a) blocks oestrogen receptors in the hypothalamus
     (b) cannot initiate gonadotrophin release if circulating levels of
          oestrogen and progesterone are high
   T (c) can be used to induce ovulation in subjects with secondary
          hypogonadism
     (d) administration carries a greater risk of ovarian
          'hyperstimulation' than gonadotrophin
     (e) should be used in the treatment of ovulatory failure only if
          gonadotrophin therapy has failed.

94 Testosterone
     (a) is secreted by the testis in response to pituitary secretion of
          FSH
     (b) stimulates gonadotrophin secretion
   T (c) may be secreted in normal amounts in seminiferous tubular
          failure
     (d) deficiency, if due to primary testicular failure, is accompanied
          by low levels of pituitary gonadotrophin
   T (e) is usually estimated in plasma by radio-immunoassay.

95 In the insulin stress test
   T (a) the object is to lower plasma glucose levels to less than
          2.5 mmol/litre and produced symptoms
   T (b) the standard dose of insulin is 0.15 U/kg body weight
     (c) if impaired pituitary function is suspected, a dose of
          0.3 U/kg should be given
   T (d) medical supervision is necessary throughout the test
     (e) if the hypoglycaemia is sufficiently severe to warrant
          intravenous glucose administration the test should be
          discontinued immediately.

Chapter VIII
Thyroid Function: TSH

96 The following statements about the synthesis of thyroid hormones
    are correct:

used F (a) Iodide uptake by the thyroid can be blocked by carbimazole.
         (b) Trapped iodide is converted to iodine in the thyroid.
         (c) Most of the tri-iodothyronine circulating in the blood is not
              formed in the thyroid.
         (d) TSH regulates the uptake of iodide.
         (e) Mono- and di-iodotyrosine are released from thyroglobulin
              at the same time as the thyroid hormones.

97 Thyroxine
         (a) does not exist in a free state in the thyroid gland
         (b) is 99 per cent protein bound in the plasma
    used (c) concentration in plasma is normally some 60—70 times that
              of tri-iodothyronine
         (d) in the unbound state in plasma is approximately equal in
              concentration to that of unbound tri-iodothyronine
    used (e) increases the sensitivity of the heart to catecholamines.

98 In the assessment of plasma levels of free thyroxine
         (a) a rise in total plasma thyroxine is accompanied by a rise in
              protein-bound and free fractions if the level of binding
              proteins remains constant
    F   (b) a rise in the level of thyroxine-binding globulin (TBG) causes
              the level of free thyroxine to fall
    used (c) with a constant level of TBG, a rise in total thyroxine causes
              a fall in the number of free binding sites
         (d) if the number of TBG binding sites is reduced, resin uptake
              of added radioactive thyroxine will be increased
    F   (e) a rise in total plasma thyroxine with a constant level of TBG
              will lead to a decreased resin uptake of added radioactive
              thyroxine.

99 The number of available thyroid-hormone binding sites on TBG
    is increased
         (a) in pregnancy
    F   (b) in the nephrotic syndrome
         (c) in women taking some oral contraceptives
    F   (d) in patients taking aspirin
         (e) in newborn babies.

100   Graves' disease
      (a)   occurs at any age
      (b)   is commoner in females
      (c)   is one of the autoimmune thyroid diseases
      (d)   is associated with exophthalmos
      (e)   is associated with multiple toxic thyroid nodules.

101   Measurement of basal plasma TSH may provide useful information
      in the diagnosis of
      (a)   Graves' disease
      (b)   toxic thyroid adenoma
      (c)   idiopathic hypothyroidism
      (d)   Hashimoto's disease
      (e)   secondary hypothyroidism.

102   A patient is strongly suspected on clinical grounds of having
      Graves' disease but the plasma total T_4 is within normal limits.
      Useful further information could be obtained by measuring
      (a)   the plasma T_3 level
      (b)   thyroid antibodies
      (c)   the plasma TSH level after TRH administration
      (d)   the plasma creatine kinase level
      (e)   the free TBG binding sites.

103   In hypothyroidism
      (a)   a plasma thyroxine within the normal range excludes the
            diagnosis
      (b)   the plasma TSH level is always raised
      (c)   due to long-standing pituitary failure, irreversible atrophic
            changes occur in the thyroid gland
      (d)   a subnormal response following TRH injection implies
            hypothalamic dysfunction
      (e)   the gland responsible is the thyroid much more commonly
            than the pituitary.

104   Neonatal hypothyroidism
   F (a)   is rarer than most inborn errors of metabolism
      (b)   must be treated in the first few months if permanent brain
            damage is to be avoided
      (c)   in the first month may be accompanied by high values of
            plasma total thyroxine
   F (d)   is characterized by low TBG levels
      (e)   is characterized by plasma TSH results which are almost
            invariably high.

105   Rarer causes of hyperthyroidism include
      (a)   secretion of thyroxine by tumours of trophoblastic origin
      (b)   lithium therapy
      (c)   ingestion of iodine by a patient with iodine deficiency goitre
      (d)   para-aminosalicylic acid therapy
      (e)   struma ovarii.

106 Characteristic features of hypothyroidism include
  (a) raised plasma creatine kinase levels
  F (b) undetectable plasma T_3 levels
  Used —— (c) raised plasma cholesterol concentration
  F (d) pretibial myxoedema
  (e) thickening of subcutaneous tissues.

Chapter IX
Carbohydrate Metabolism and Its Interrelationships

107 The following are reducing sugars:
- (a) fructose
- (b) galactose
- (c) sucrose
- (d) maltose
- (e) lactose.

108 Hepatic mechanisms involved in regulating the level of plasma glucose include
- (a) synthesis of glycogen from glucose-6-phosphate
- (b) conversion of glucose to amino acids
- (c) conversion of glycogen to glucose
- (d) active transport of glucose from plasma to liver cells under the influence of insulin
- (e) conversion of glucose to fatty acids.

109 Actions of insulin include
- (a) stimulation of glycogenolysis by the liver
- (b) induction of the hepatic enzyme responsible for the conversion of glucose to glucose-6-phosphate
- (c) stimulation of entry of glucose into brain cells
- (d) stimulation of entry of glucose into adipose tissue
- (e) stimulation of glycogenesis in muscle.

110 The following mechanisms play a recognized part in fat metabolism:
- (a) conversion of adipose tissue triglyceride to free fatty acids and glycerol during fasting
- (b) conversion of free fatty acid to glycogen in muscles during fasting
- (c) utilization of ketoacids by brain tissue as an energy source during prolonged fasting
- (d) conversion in adipose tissue of excess glucose to triglyceride
- (e) generation of fatty acids from acetyl coenzyme A in the liver.

111 Lactic acidosis can occur as a result of
- (a) strenuous exercise
- (b) cardiac arrest
- (c) administration of phenformin
- (d) leukaemia
- (e) glucose-6-phosphatase deficiency (von Gierke's disease).

112 Glucagon promotes
    (a) hepatic gluconeogenesis
    (b) glucose uptake by muscle
    (c) glycogen synthesis by muscle
    (d) breakdown of protein
    (e) synthesis of fat.

113 Effects of glucocorticoids on carbohydrate metabolism include:
    (a) promotion of hepatic gluconeogenesis
    (b) suppression of uptake of glucose by muscles
    (c) promotion of protein breakdown
    (d) promotion of fat breakdown
    (e) promotion of glycogen breakdown by the liver.

114 Secretion of insulin is stimulated by
    (a) hyperglycaemia
    (b) some amino acids
    (c) glucagon
    (d) adrenaline (epinephrine)
    (e) fasting.

115 Glycosuria detectable by side-room tests
    (a) always requires further investigation
    (b) usually occurs at plasma glucose levels higher than
        7.0 mmol/litre
    (c) always indicates hyperglycaemia
    (d) may be absent in circulatory insufficiency even with severe
        hyperglycaemia
    (e) is best detected by enzyme reagent strips.

116 Non-insulin-dependent diabetes mellitus
    (a) is the commonest variety of diabetes
    (b) may need insulin treatment
    (c) rarely proceeds to ketoacidosis
    (d) is frequently controlled by diet and weight reduction
    (e) may be associated with high plasma insulin levels.

117 Hypoglycaemia
    (a) is uncommon in infancy
    (b) is of little importance in the first few months of life
    (c) occurs in about 10 per cent of babies of diabetic mothers
    (d) due to von Gierke's disease is best treated by infusion of
        fructose
    (e) is present at birth in galactosaemia.

118   In the investigation of suspected diabetes mellitus
    (a) random plasma glucose levels are most useful in *excluding* the diagnosis
    (b) fasting plasma glucose levels of over 8 mmol/litre need to be followed up by a glucose tolerance test
    (c) the WHO classifies patients with a plasma glucose of 8–11 mmol/litre two hours after a 75 g glucose load as having impaired glucose tolerance
    (d) most patients with impaired glucose tolerance later develop diabetes mellitus
    (e) a glucose tolerance test will distinguish between insulin-dependent and non-insulin-dependent types of diabetes.

119   Diabetes may be associated with
    (a) haemochromatosis
    (b) acromegaly
    (c) hypopituitarism
    (d) treatment with chlorothiazide
    (e) chronic pancreatitis.

120   In insulin-dependent diabetes
    (a) symptoms usually appear after the age of 40
    (b) there is an absolute insulin deficiency
    (c) there is a substantial risk of ketoacidosis and coma
    (d) a relationship with specific HLA tissue types has been identified
    (e) obesity is usual.

121   Biochemical abnormalities associated with insulin-dependent diabetes include
    (a) increased breakdown of protein
    (b) depressed levels of plasma free fatty acids
    (c) increased synthesis of cholesterol
    (d) increased chylomicrons in peripheral blood
    (e) increase in plasma low-density lipoprotein.

122   In the diagnosis of diabetes mellitus the following should be borne in mind:
    (a) Glucose normally appears in the urine when the plasma level rises above 11 mmol/litre.
    (b) An early morning specimen of urine is the most reliable.
    (c) In the presence of a reduced glomerular filtration rate the renal threshold may be lowered.
    (d) A fasting plasma glucose level of more than 8 mmol/litre is almost diagnostic of diabetes.
    (e) A fasting plasma glucose level consistently below 6 mmol/litre rules out the diagnosis of diabetes.

123 When using simple urine tests it should be remembered that
 (a) glucose may be present in the urine when plasma levels are normal
 (b) false negative results for glucose may be obtained if the patient is taking ascorbic acid supplements
 (c) most tests for ketones detect only β-hydroxybutyrate
 (d) in Rothera's test a purple-red colour indicates that ketones are present
 (e) a fast must go on for several days before ketonuria is detectable.

124 The following conditions occurring in a diabetic tend to increase the patient's insulin requirement
 (a) pregnancy
 (b) Addison's disease
 (c) acromegaly
 (d) infection
 (e) trauma.

125 The following laboratory results would be adequately explained by the diagnosis of diabetic ketoacidosis:
 (a) plasma total osmolarity 345 mmol/litre
 (b) plasma total CO_2 9 mmol/litre
 (c) plasma urea 2.0 mmol/litre
 (d) blood haemoglobin 18.0 g/dl
 (e) plasma amylase four times the upper limit of normal.

126 In hyperosmolal non-ketotic coma
 (a) the patient is usually elderly
 (b) hyperventilation does not occur
 (c) plasma glucose levels of up to 50 mmol/litre are not uncommon
 (d) the cause of the coma is thought to be cerebral dehydration
 (e) resistance to insulin is a typical feature.

127 The following usually need to be given intravenously during the treatment of diabetic ketoacidosis
 (a) isotonic saline
 (b) a large bolus of insulin
 (c) potassium chloride
 (d) hypertonic saline
 (e) 16.8 per cent sodium bicarbonate.

128 Recognized causes of hypoglycaemia include
 (a) salicylate poisoning
 (b) insulinoma
 (c) Addison's disease
 (d) severe liver disease
 (e) retroperitoneal sarcoma.

129   Alcohol-induced hypoglycaemia
    (a)   is commoner when there has been antecedent starvation
    (b)   is thought to be due to suppression of hepatic
         gluconeogenesis
    (c)   is always easily distinguished from alcoholic stupor on
         clinical grounds alone
    (d)   rarely needs to be treated with glucose infusion
    (e)   is difficult to reproduce by infusion of alcohol unless the
         patient has fasted for some time previously.

130   A patient is found to develop hypoglycaemia with some
    regularity between three and four hours after a carbohydrate
    meal. This history is compatible with the following diseases:
    (a)   previous gastrectomy
    (b)   insulinoma
    (c)   chronic aspirin ingestion
    (d)   chronic liver disease
    (e)   functional reactive hypoglycaemia.

131   In a patient with an insulinoma
    (a)   C-peptide levels are suppressed
    (b)   symptoms are most common two hours after meals
    (c)   symptoms are sporadic
    (d)   the tumour involves the β-cells of the pancreas
    (e)   metastasis commonly occurs.

132   In interpreting the results of plasma glucose measurements the
    following points need to be kept in mind:
    (a)   Enzymatic methods tend to give a result lower than the true
         glucose value.
    (b)   Whole blood glucose values may be 10–15 per cent lower
         than those obtained from measurements on plasma or serum.
    (c)   Release of glucose from cells may cause erroneously high
         values to be recorded on blood which has been collected into
         the wrong anticoagulant.
    (d)   Capillary blood tends to give higher glucose levels than
         venous blood.
    (e)   Methods measuring total reducing substances are most
         reliable at low levels of glucose.

133   The following statements about tests for sugar in the urine are
    correct:
    (a)   The Clinistix test is more sensitive than Clinitest tablets.
    (b)   Clinistix gives a positive result for glucose and for no other
         sugar.
    (c)   Clinitest tablets are better suited than Clinistix to semi-
         quantitative estimation of urine glucose.
    (d)   When screening tests are being performed on urine from
         neonates or babies, Clinitest is preferable to Clinistix.
    (e)   A positive result with Clinitest in an adult may be due to the
         ingestion of aspirin.

134 The oral glucose tolerance test as recommended by the WHO
    (a) must be preceded by three to four days of dietary carbohydrate restriction
    (b) is best performed in the morning
    (c) may be performed using a mixture of glucose and its oligosaccharides
    (d) involves venous blood sampling every half hour for two hours
    (e) should be preceded by a 10–16 hour fast.

135 In the management of severe diabetic ketoacidosis
    (a) initial assessment should be made and therapy begun on the basis of the clinical findings without waiting for laboratory results
    (b) the results of urine testing for glucose give a reliable assessment of the patient's status
    (c) the results of testing the patient's blood with a reagent strip may be dangerously fallacious
    (d) the arterial blood pH should be measured frequently
    (e) plasma ketone levels should be measured in every case.

136 The planning of intravenous feeding should be based on the following:
    (a) If food intake is withdrawn, hepatic glycogen stores will last for some 7–10 days.
    (b) Infusion of 40 per cent glucose into a peripheral vein is likely to cause thrombosis.
    (c) The infusion of fat emulsions should be interrupted for a few hours before blood sampling for biochemical analysis.
    (d) 20 per cent emulsions of fat may be infused into peripheral veins with very little risk of thrombosis.
    (e) Amino acid infusion during the catabolic phase is likely to be ineffective.

Chapter X
Plasma Lipids and Lipoproteins

137 The following statements about the lipids present in plasma are
correct:
   (a) Palmitic acid contains no double bonds.
   (b) Most fatty acids are branched-chain compounds.
   (c) Free fatty acids are an immediately available energy source.
   (d) Free fatty acids are carried mainly bound to albumin.
   (e) About two-thirds of the plasma cholesterol is combined with
       glycerol.

138 All lipoproteins contain
   (a) cholesterol
   (b) phospholipids
   (c) free fatty acids
   (d) triglycerides
   (e) apoproteins.

139 In correlating the electrophoretic characteristics of plasma lipids
with their behaviour on ultracentrifugation and their chemical
composition, the following statements are correct:
   (a) Pre-β lipoproteins correspond with the VLDL fraction.
   (b) α lipoproteins correspond with the LDL fraction.
   (c) α lipoproteins contain the highest proportion of protein.
   (d) Chylomicrons are largely composed of triglycerides.
   (e) β lipoproteins contain the highest proportion of cholesterol.

140 Chylomicrons
   (a) are not normally present in plasma in the fasting state
   (b) are passed intact from the intestinal lumen via the intestinal
       cells to the blood
   (c) are metabolized principally by adipose tissue and muscle
   (d) are responsible for the turbidity of plasma after a fatty meal
   (e) after hydrolysis by lipoprotein lipase yield remnant particles
       consisting mainly of phospholipid.

141 The following statements concerning the metabolism of
endogenous lipids are correct:
   (a) Given a high carbohydrate intake, the liver is capable of
       synthesizing FFA from glucose.
   (b) The sole site of cholesterol synthesis is the liver.
   (c) Endogenous cholesterol and triglyceride are transported from
       the liver as HDL.
   (d) Endogenous triglycerides are hydrolysed by lipoprotein
       lipase on the capillary wall.
   (e) Endogenous synthesis of cholesterol is suppressed by cellular
       uptake of LDL.

142 High-density lipoprotein
   (a) is essential for the transport of cholesterol from the peripheral tissues to the liver
   (b) contains little or no phospholipid
   (c) in the fasting subject contains most of the apoprotein C found in plasma
   (d) transports cholesterol as macromolecular complexes of the non-esterified lipid
   (e) contains 80—90 per cent of the triglyceride in plasma.

143 The following factors influence the level of plasma cholesterol in the ways described:
   (a) A large increase in dietary cholesterol causes an exactly equivalent decrease in hepatic cholesterol synthesis so that the plasma cholesterol level remains unaltered.
   (b) An increase in dietary saturated fatty acids leads to higher plasma cholesterol levels.
   (c) An increase in dietary polyunsaturated fatty acids leads to lower plasma cholesterol levels.
   (d) Cholesterol excreted in the bile is available for reabsorption.
   (e) Administration of cholestyramine is effective in reducing plasma cholesterol levels.

144 The level of plasma HDL cholesterol
   (a) is negatively correlated with the risk of cardiovascular disease
   (b) is lower in women of reproductive age than in men
   (c) tends to rise as a result of physical exercise
   (d) tends to rise if the diet is rich in carbohydrate
   (e) is reduced in Tangier disease.

145 In the assessment of possible hyperlipidaemia the following considerations must be borne in mind:
   (a) Plasma triglyceride levels rise significantly after a meal containing fat.
   (b) Plasma cholesterol levels are only slightly affected by a meal containing fat.
   (c) Plasma cholesterol at birth is usually below 2.6 mmol/litre (100 mg/dl).
   (d) Plasma cholesterol in affluent societies may rise at least as high as 8.4 mmol/litre (330 mg/dl) in the fifth and sixth decades.
   (e) Plasma cholesterol levels rise transiently above the adult level at puberty.

146 Recognized causes of hyperlipidaemia include
   (a) hyperthyroidism
   (b) biliary obstruction
   (c) alcohol abuse
   (d) diabetes mellitus
   (e) pregnancy.

147   Blood is drawn into an EDTA tube from a fasting patient with
       suspected hyperlipidaemia and separated by centrifugation. The
       fresh plasma is turbid to the naked eye. After 18 hours
       at 4°C the appearance is unchanged. The following conclusions
       may be drawn:
       (a) The plasma triglyceride level is almost certainly raised.
       (b) There is clear evidence of increased LDL levels.
       (c) A history of the ingestion of oral contraceptives could
            explain the findings.
       (d) The presence of hyperuricaemia would be consistent with
            the findings.
       (e) Treatment with cholestyramine is indicated.

148   In familial (monogenic) hypercholesterolaemia
       (a) there is autosomal dominant inheritance
       (b) homozygotes rarely survive beyond the age of 20
       (c) heterozygotes have a normal life expectancy
       (d) plasma triglyceride levels are usually normal
       (e) tendinous xanthomata do not occur in heterozygotes until the
            second decade or later.

149   Polygenic hypercholesterolaemia
       (a) is so called because, in affected families, there is a continuous
            distribution of plasma cholesterol levels with a higher than
            normal mean value
       (b) is unaffected by the composition of the diet
       (c) involves an increased risk of cardiovascular disease
       (d) should not be diagnosed unless xanthomata can be
            demonstrated
       (e) is usually associated with a turbid plasma.

150   In familial endogenous hypertriglyceridaemia
       (a) transmission is probably as an autosomal dominant trait
       (b) clinical manifestations appear in the first year of life
       (c) there is an increase in plasma VLDL
       (d) hyperchylomicronaemia may be present
       (e) there is a recognized association with glucose intolerance.

151   In familial combined hyperlipidaemia
       (a) there is reduced production of apoprotein B in the liver
       (b) the plasma triglyceride level may be normal
       (c) the lipid abnormalities only become apparent after the third
            decade
       (d) eruptive xanthomata may be found
       (e) there is no increased risk of cardiovascular disease.

152   The following items of advice are appropriate in hyperlipidaemia:
    (a)   Carbohydrate intake should be restricted in endogenous hypertriglyceridaemia.
    (b)   Animal fats should be avoided in hypercholesterolaemia.
    (c)   Intake of fat in all forms should be restricted in exogenous hypertriglyceridaemia.
    (d)   Intake of alcohol should be restricted in all forms of hyperlipidaemia.
    (e)   Dietary measures alone are the recommended treatment for familial (monogenic) hypercholesterolaemia.

Chapter XI
Calcium, Phosphate and Magnesium Metabolism

153 The intestinal absorption of calcium is
    (a) decreased in renal failure
    (b) usually 25—50 per cent of dietary intake
    (c) increased by the oral intake of phosphate
    (d) increased by 1, 25-dihydroxycholecalciferol
    (e) decreased in the presence of steatorrhoea.

154 Parathyroid hormone
    (a) is released through the action of the parathyroid stimulating hormone of the anterior pituitary
    (b) requires vitamin D in physiological amounts for its effective action
    (c) acts on bone by stimulation of the osteoclasts
    (d) has an action on the plasma calcium level opposite to that of calcitonin
    (e) decreases the urinary excretion of phosphate.

155 Cholecalciferol
    (a) may be formed in the skin by the action of ultraviolet light
    (b) is found in the free form in plasma
    (c) in adults is derived mainly from dietary intake
    (d) is hydroxylated to 25-hydroxycholecalciferol in the liver
    (e) given orally in adequate dosage will restore a low plasma calcium concentration to normal in 24 hours.

156 Hypercalcaemia is a recognized consequence of
    (a) excessive secretion of calcitonin
    (b) excessive secretion of thyroid hormone
    (c) malignant disease
    (d) secondary hyperparathyroidism
    (e) sarcoidosis.

157 Recognized consequences of hypercalcaemia include
    (a) polyuria
    (b) diarrhoea
    (c) cardiac arrest
    (d) nausea
    (e) cataract.

158   The following would be consistent with a diagnosis of long-
      standing primary hyperparathyroidism:
      (a) a greatly elevated plasma alkaline phosphatase
      (b) pseudo-fractures on X-ray
      (c) subperiosteal erosions on X-ray
      (d) uncalcified osteoid in a bone biopsy
      (e) evidence of renal functional impairment.

159   In tertiary hyperparathyroidism
      (a) the plasma alkaline phosphatase level is usually normal
      (b) the plasma calcium is usually low at the time of diagnosis
      (c) the plasma level of parathyroid hormone is raised
      (d) an ectopic source of parathyroid hormone is present
      (e) urinary phosphate excretion is increased if renal function is
           unimpaired.

160   Recognized causes of secondary hyperparathyroidism include
      (a) malnutrition
      (b) steatorrhoea
      (c) Fanconi syndrome
      (d) renal failure
      (e) administration of anticonvulsants.

161   A patient is found to have a plasma calcium of 2.90 mmol/litre and
      a plasma inorganic phosphate of 0.70 mmol/litre. These findings
      are compatible with a diagnosis of
      (a) Paget's disease of bone
      (b) osteoporosis
      (c) malabsorption syndrome
      (d) a parathyroid adenoma
      (e) advanced renal failure.

162   Hypoparathyroidism
      (a) is a recognized cause of depression
      (b) is an almost inevitable consequence of total thyroidectomy
      (c) can be due to primary atrophy of the glands
      (d) may cause visual impairment
      (e) is associated with a high incidence of peptic ulceration.

163   A man of 30 is found to have a plasma calcium level of
      3.00 mmol/litre; his plasma PTH level is below the limit of
      detection. These findings may be due to
      (a) sarcoidosis
      (b) advanced renal failure
      (c) myelomatosis
      (d) thyrotoxicosis
      (e) intestinal malabsorption.

164   Sensitivity to the action of vitamin D is thought to be increased in
    (a)   renal damage
    (b)   idiopathic hypercalcaemia of infancy
    (c)   sarcoidosis
    (d)   thyrotoxicosis
    (e)   chronic liver disease.

165   A rise in total plasma calcium without any change in the ionized fraction could be due to
    (a)   prolonged stasis during venepuncture
    (b)   malnutrition
    (c)   acute pancreatitis
    (d)   dehydration of the patient
    (e)   hyperventilation by the patient.

166   In a patient with hypercalcaemia of undetermined origin, the administration of steroids will nearly always restore the plasma calcium to normal if the patient has
    (a)   primary hyperparathyroidism
    (b)   vitamin D intoxication
    (c)   tertiary hyperparathyroidism
    (d)   ectopic PTH production
    (e)   myelomatosis.

167   Increased urinary excretion of calcium is a recognized feature of
    (a)   actively progressing osteoporosis
    (b)   renal tubular acidosis
    (c)   renal glomerular failure
    (d)   thyrotoxicosis
    (e)   secondary hyperparathyroidism.

168   The level of plasma phosphate is usually reduced below normal in
    (a)   vitamin D deficiency
    (b)   hypoparathyroidism
    (c)   acromegaly
    (d)   renal glomerular failure
    (e)   vitamin D resistant rickets.

169   In the case of a patient with a plasma calcium level of 4.00 mmol/litre, effective control could be achieved within a few hours by
    (a)   inducing a water diuresis
    (b)   administering hydrocortisone orally
    (c)   administering sodium phosphate orally
    (d)   administering sodium phosphate intravenously
    (e)   administering calcitonin intramuscularly.

170 Hypocalcaemia
(a) following removal of a parathyroid adenoma should be treated as soon as it is detected
(b) in renal failure should only be treated after giving oral aluminium hydroxide
(c) is easily treated in asymptomatic cases with oral calcium supplements
(d) causing tetany may be treated with intravenous calcium gluconate
(e) treated with calciferol is more likely to result in ectopic calcification than treatment with 1, 25-DHCC.

171 Recognized causes of hypomagnesaemia include
(a) diarrhoea
(b) renal glomerular failure
(c) hypoparathyroidism
(d) primary aldosteronism
(e) diuretic therapy.

Chapter XII
Intestinal Absorption: Pancreatic and Gastric Function

172   The following statements are correct:
   (a)   About 90 per cent of the water entering the gastro-intestinal tract is reabsorbed in the colon.
   (b)   Disturbances of hydrogen ion homeostasis are an important complication of malabsorption syndromes.
   (c)   Quantitatively the most important digestion occurs in the lower jejunum and ileum.
   (d)   Most fluid entering the gastro-intestinal tract is derived from plasma by passive ultrafiltration.
   (e)   In health dietary fat is almost completely absorbed.

173   Intestinal absorption
   (a)   of dietary glucose depends on intact pancreatic function
   (b)   of vitamin B_{12} requires its previous digestion by intrinsic factor
   (c)   of fats is accomplished largely by the transport of chylomicrons from the intestinal lumen to the blood
   (d)   of fat-soluble vitamins may be impaired as a result of the administration of broad-spectrum antibiotics
   (e)   of unhydrolysed oligosaccharides does not normally occur.

174   Bile salts
   (a)   emulsify fat entering the duodenum
   (b)   potentiate the activity of pancreatic lipase
   (c)   are re-absorbed in the distal ileum
   (d)   aggregate with lipids to form micelles
   (e)   can be deconjugated in the bowel lumen by some intestinal bacteria.

175   Naturally occurring triglycerides
   (a)   contain glycerol combined with three identical fatty acid molecules
   (b)   are not present in micelles
   (c)   are resynthesised in intestinal cells
   (d)   are hydrolysed by pancreatic lipase mainly to 2-monoglycerides and free fatty acids
   (e)   are not present in chylomicrons.

176   Cholesterol
   (a)   is present in micelles in esterified form
   (b)   is synthesized from bile salts in the liver
   (c)   is re-esterified in the intestinal cells
   (d)   esters contain either glycine or taurine
   (e)   in esterified form is present in chylomicrons.

177   The following substances are absorbed intact into the portal
       circulation:
       (a)   amino acids
       (b)   most small peptides
       (c)   some free fatty acids
       (d)   vitamin K
       (e)   monosaccharides.

178   Enzymes present on the brush border of the intestinal cells
       include
       (a)   maltase
       (b)   lactase
       (c)   peptidase
       (d)   sucrase
       (e)   amylase.

179   The following statements about carbohydrate digestion and
       absorption are correct:
       (a)   Starch is hydrolysed to disaccharides by salivary and
             pancreatic amylase.
       (b)   Sucrose, maltose and lactose all contain glucose.
       (c)   Monosaccharides are absorbed in the duodenum.
       (d)   The two constituent monosaccharides of sucrose are
             probably absorbed by a common active process.
       (e)   A significant proportion of absorbed carbohydrate originates
             from intestinal secretions and desquamated mucosal cells.

180   The intestinal absorption of
       (a)   calcium takes place mainly in the upper small intestine
       (b)   iron is stimulated by anaemia
       (c)   magnesium probably requires the presence of vitamin D
       (d)   vitamin B_{12} is mainly in the duodenum and upper jejunum
       (e)   calcium is enhanced by the presence of a high concentration of
             fatty acids in the intestine.

181   Recognized causes of *generalized* malabsorption include
       (a)   blind-loop syndrome
       (b)   biliary obstruction
       (c)   carcinoid syndrome
       (d)   tropical sprue
       (e)   idiopathic steatorrhoea.

182   Coeliac disease
       (a)   can be distinguished from tropical sprue by the findings on
             intestinal biopsy
       (b)   occurs at any age
       (c)   responds to treatment with a diet from which wheat germ
             has been excluded
       (d)   is a recognized cause of osteoporosis
       (e)   requires treatment with broad-spectrum antibiotics in
             addition to modification of the diet.

183 Fibrocystic disease of the pancreas
(a) is a likely diagnosis if the sweat sodium concentration is about half normal
(b) is a recognized complication of chronic pancreatitis
(c) causes malabsorption predominantly of all forms of carbohydrate
(d) has a recognized association with chronic pulmonary disease
(e) is characterized by a marked elevation in plasma amylase levels.

184 Recognized clinical manifestations of severe prolonged generalized malabsorption include
(a) pale bulky stools
(b) tetany
(c) muscle wasting
(d) recurrent infections
(e) oedema.

185 Recognized laboratory findings in idiopathic steatorrhoea include
(a) hypocalcaemia
(b) hyperphosphataemia
(c) a raised alkaline phosphatase in cases with osteomalacia
(d) a low plasma trypsin level
(e) prolonged prothrombin time.

186 It may be possible to distinguish malabsorption due to pancreatic disease from generalized intestinal malabsorption because in the former
(a) malabsorption of fat does not occur
(b) the Lundh test is likely to be normal
(c) xylose absorption is normal
(d) intestinal biopsy is likely to be normal
(e) anaemia is more common.

187 Recognized consequences of gastric resection include
(a) a reduction in the efficiency of enzyme action in the small intestine
(b) hypoglycaemia about 30 minutes after a meal
(c) a reduction in plasma volume after a meal
(d) mild malabsorption
(e) dilatation of the duodenum after a meal by a large volume of fluid.

188 Acute pancreatitis
(a) should not be diagnosed if the plasma amylase level is normal
(b) is commonly the result of obstruction of the pancreatic duct
(c) is typically associated with levels of plasma amylase higher than those seen in any other acute abdominal emergency
(d) may be precipitated by hypertriglyceridaemia
(e) may be due to trauma to the pancreas.

189   Alteration of the bacterial flora in the intestine typically causes
      (a)   iron deficiency anaemia
      (b)   steatorrhoea
      (c)   jaundice
      (d)   impaired absorption of xylose
      (e)   hypoalbuminaemia.

190   In the investigation of megaloblastic anaemia
      (a)   a Schilling test should precede examination of the bone-
            marrow
      (b)   a history of total gastrectomy suggests that the oral
            administration of intrinsic factor will restore the absorption
            of vitamin B_{12} to normal
      (c)   the absorption of vitamin B_{12} is uninfluenced by the oral
            administration of intrinsic factor in Crohn's disease
      (d)   the finding of antibodies to parietal cells and to intrinsic
            factor is in favour of a diagnosis of pernicious anaemia
      (e)   a large oral dose of non-radioactive vitamin B_{12} should be
            given together with the radioactive vitamin in the Schilling test.

191   Disaccharidase deficiency
      (a)   causes symptoms similar to those of the 'dumping syndrome'
      (b)   is a recognized feature of generalized intestinal malabsorption
      (c)   is typically associated with alkaline stools
      (d)   is most reliably diagnosed by estimation of the relevant
            enzymes in intestinal biopsy tissue
      (e)   produces abnormalities in a barium meal if the relevant
            disaccharide is administered with the barium.

192   Lactase deficiency
      (a)   is more often congenital than acquired
      (b)   in premature infants is usually a transient disorder
      (c)   of the congenital type causes severe constipation in the
            neonatal period
      (d)   usually coexists with isomaltase deficiency
      (e)   is common in the Chinese.

193   Protein-losing enteropathy
      (a)   is usually associated with steatorrhoea
      (b)   is a recognized cause of oedema
      (c)   can be diagnosed by measuring the loss into the bowel of
            parenteral radioactive polyvinylpyrrolidone
      (d)   typically causes a predominant loss of α_2-globulins into the
            bowel
      (e)   may be due to obstruction of the lymphatics draining the
            bowel.

194 The following statements about gastric secretion are correct:
   (a) The sight, smell or taste of food stimulate gastric secretion via the vagus nerve.
   (b) Gastrin is secreted in the gastric antrum.
   (c) Acid in the pylorus inhibits the secretion of gastrin.
   (d) Antihistamines and cimetidine have similar effects on gastric secretion.
   (e) Gastrin acts mainly on the gastric antrum.

195 Recognized features of the Zollinger—Ellison syndrome include
   (a) a very high basal gastric acid secretion
   (b) a greater than normal gastric acid secretion in response to pentagastrin
   (c) duodenal ulceration
   (d) diarrhoea
   (e) steatorrhoea.

Chapter XIII
Liver Disease and Gall Stones

196 The following substances are normally synthesized in the liver:
   (a) glucose
   (b) vitamin K
   (c) triglycerides
   (d) immunoglobulins
   (e) prothrombin.

197 Fatty acids reaching the liver from the fat stores may be
   (a) converted to glucose
   (b) conjugated with sulphate
   (c) metabolized in the tricarboxylic acid cycle
   (d) incorporated into endogenous triglyceride
   (e) converted into ketones.

198 The breakdown of circulating red cells
   (a) takes place mainly in the Kupffer cells of the liver
   (b) leads to the release of haemoglobin from which globin is
        split and enters the general protein pool
   (c) is followed by the removal from haem of iron which is
        largely excreted in the urine
   (d) is not the only source of the bilirubin reaching the liver
   (e) normally produces about 400 μmol of bilirubin daily.

199 Unconjugated bilirubin
   (a) is normally present in the plasma in lower concentration
        than conjugated bilirubin
   (b) normally circulates in the plasma bound to albumin
   (c) is not excreted in the urine
   (d) is displaced from protein by salicylates
   (e) is bound to specific proteins in the liver cells.

200 The conjugation of bilirubin
   (a) takes place at the smooth endoplasmic reticulum
   (b) is catalysed by the enzyme uridyl diphosphate (UDP)
        glucuronyl transferase
   (c) may be inhibited by anions
   (d) renders it water-soluble
   (e) is impaired in the Dubin—Johnson syndrome.

201 Urobilinogen
   (a) is colourless
   (b) is never detectable in normal urine
   (c) is produced by the bacterial breakdown of stercobilinogen
   (d) is present in large amounts in the urine in acute haemolytic
        states
   (e) can be oxidized to a coloured compound.

202   Recognized causes of intrahepatic cholestasis include
(a) paracetamol therapy
(b) viral hepatitis
(c) oral contraceptive therapy
(d) xanthomatosis
(e) primary biliary cirrhosis.

203   In the liver
(a) cholesterol is excreted only after conversion to bile acids
(b) the carboxyl groups of amino acids are converted to urea
(c) steroid hormones are inactivated by conjugation with
        glucuronate and sulphate
(d) toxic substances are extracted by Kupffer cells in the hepatic
        sinusoids
(e) VLDL is synthesized.

204   Aspartate transaminase
(a) is not present in mitochondria
(b) levels in the plasma are relatively higher than those of alanine
        transaminase in hepatitis
(c) has a longer half-life than alanine transaminase
(d) levels in the plasma are relatively lower than those of alanine
        transaminase in the presence of hepatic space-occupying
        lesions
(e) levels in the plasma are not raised in cholestasis.

205   In cholestasis
(a) there is increased synthesis of alkaline phosphatase at the
        sinusoidal surface of the hepatocyte
(b) malabsorption of fat may occur
(c) plasma cholesterol levels may fall
(d) plasma alkaline phosphatase levels are highest in extra-
        hepatic obstruction
(e) raised levels of bilirubin in the plasma may cause severe
        itching.

206   In the investigation of hepatocellular function
(a) shortening of a prolonged prothrombin time after vitamin K
        injection suggests cholestasis rather than liver-cell damage
(b) a history of exposure to chlorinated hydrocarbons is relevant
(c) the highest levels of plasma transaminases are seen in chronic
        liver disease
(d) a rapid fall in very high transaminase levels is not necessarily
        a favourable prognostic sign
(e) the relative plasma activities of AST and ALT may indicate
        the nature of the damage.

207   The following statements are correct:
    (a)   The finding of antibodies to hepatitis A in the serum is strong evidence of active infection.
    (b)   Predominant elevation of serum IgG is compatible with chronic active hepatitis.
    (c)   Circulating antibodies to smooth muscle are often found in alcoholic cirrhosis.
    (d)   The finding of α-fetoprotein in serum is pathognomonic of primary hepatocellular carcinoma.
    (e)   A gamma-glutamyltransferase level raised out of proportion to the transaminase and bilirubin levels is suggestive evidence of acute alcoholic hepatitis.

208   In acute viral hepatitis
    (a)   plasma transaminase levels are invariably elevated
    (b)   with jaundice both unconjugated and conjugated plasma bilirubin levels usually rise
    (c)   the plasma alanine transaminase level falls to normal before the aspartate transaminase
    (d)   hypoalbuminaemia is an almost constant finding
    (e)   plasma alkaline phosphatase levels vary from normal to very high.

209   In a patient with clinical and biochemical evidence of prolonged biliary obstruction
    (a)   elevation of the plasma transaminase levels would prove that the cholestasis was intrahepatic
    (b)   a predominant increase in serum IgM favours a diagnosis of primary biliary cirrhosis
    (c)   the urine is likely to contain unconjugated bilirubin
    (d)   jaundice that is painless and progressive is likely to be due to a malignant obstruction
    (e)   a positive mitochondrial antibody test is in favour of primary biliary cirrhosis.

210   Typical laboratory findings in hepatic cirrhosis include
    (a)   very high plasma transaminase levels
    (b)   hypoalbuminaemia
    (c) β-γ fusion on serum protein electrophoresis
    (d)   a prolonged prothrombin time
    (e)   hyponatraemia unless ascites is present.

211   The finding of a pathologically low plasma concentration of the following substances is a recognized feature of hepatocellular failure
    (a)   glucose
    (b)   potassium
    (c)   prothrombin
    (d)   amino acids
    (e)   urea.

212 Jaundice in the neonatal period
   (a) does not require treatment unless it is due to haemolytic disease of the newborn
   (b) is more likely to lead to kernicterus if the baby is given salicylates
   (c) may be treated with novobiocin
   (d) when caused by the Crigler–Najjar syndrome is harmless
   (e) is more likely to cause brain damage if glucuronyl transferase is being induced.

213 The following statements about congenital hyperbilirubinaemia are correct:
   (a) The probable cause of the Crigler– Najjar syndrome is a deficiency of glucuronyl transferase.
   (b) The Dubin–Johnson syndrome is a recognized cause of kernicterus.
   (c) Bilirubin is not found in the urine in Gilbert's disease.
   (d) In some patients, the hyperbilirubinaemia of the Crigler–Najjar syndrome can be reduced by phenobarbitone.
   (e) The Dubin–Johnson syndrome can be diagnosed by liver biopsy.

214 Recognized causes of acute hepatic necrosis include
   (a) chlorpromazine
   (b) ferrous sulphate
   (c) paracetamol
   (d) halothane
   (e) isoniazid.

215 Bile salts
   (a) as present in the stools are the sodium salts of deoxycholic acid and lithocholic acid
   (b) as present in the bile are salts of cholic acid and chenode-oxycholic acid only
   (c) are conjugated with glucuronic acid
   (d) are present in micelles with their polar groups on the outside
   (e) are the major anions of gall bladder bile.

216 The concentration of the following substances is much higher in gall bladder bile than in hepatic bile:
   (a) conjugated bilirubin
   (b) bicarbonate
   (c) cholesterol
   (d) chloride
   (e) bile salts.

217 Gall stones
 (a) are more often radio-opaque than are renal calculi
 (b) with a crystalline appearance on the cut surface probably
      consist of cholesterol
 (c) are particularly common in patients with hypercholester-
      olaemia
 (d) are usually multiple
 (e) are most commonly of the mixed type.

218 The following statements are true of gall stones:
 (a) Pigment stones are associated with chronic haemolytic states.
 (b) Stones occur in all patients with a high concentration of
      cholesterol in their bile.
 (c) A high total concentration of bile salts is a predisposing
      factor.
 (d) The incidence is increased by oral contraceptive preparations.
 (e) It is important to analyse all gall stones chemically.

219 When testing the urine for bile pigments and their derivatives with
     reagent strips
 (a) a positive test for urobilinogen should be confirmed by a
      test for urobilin
 (b) chlorpromazine may give a false positive reaction for
      urobilinogen
 (c) fresh urine is essential
 (d) Urobilistix may detect urobilinogen in some urines from
      normal subjects
 (e) Urobilistix reacts with both urobilinogen and porpho-
      bilinogen.

Chapter XIV
Proteins in Plasma and Urine

220 Plasma proteins
  (a) which combine with drugs enhance their pharmacological activity
  T (b) of low molecular weight are passively lost through the glomerulus under physiological conditions
  T (c) which combine with lipids render them water-soluble
  T (d) affect the distribution of water between intra- and extra-vascular compartments
  (e) are normally in a concentration of about 7g/litre.

221 Recognized causes of hyperalbuminaemia include
  (a) stasis during venepuncture
  (b) dehydration
  (c) severe burns
  (d) auto-immune disease
  (e) bisalbuminaemia.

222 The serum albumin concentration
  (a) may fall by a small amount as a result of apparently minor illness
  (b) typically rises during late pregnancy
  (c) is higher in the upright than in the recumbent position
  (d) can be assumed to be normal if the total protein concentration is normal
  (e) is typically below normal in extensive psoriasis.

223 Recognized consequences of hypoalbuminaemia include
  T (a) hypocalcaemia
  T (b) an increased risk of toxic effects in patients on sulphon-amides
  T (c) oedema
  T (d) potentiation of the bactericidal effect of penicillin
  (e) tetany.

224

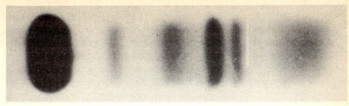

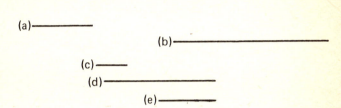

(a)————————

(b)——————————————————

(c)——————

(d)————————————

(e)——————————

In the electrophoretic strip shown above the positions of the following proteins are correctly lettered:
- (a) albumin
- (b) IgG
- (c) α_1-antitrypsin
- (d) IgM
- (e) β-lipoprotein.

225 The following proteins have molecular weights lower than that of albumin:
- (a) IgG
- (b) Bence Jones protein
- (c) α_1-antitrypsin
- (d) IgA
- (e) cryoglobulins

226 The α_2-globulin fraction
- (a) is characteristically in high relative or absolute concentration in the serum in the nephrotic syndrome
- (b) falls in concentration in the serum as a non-specific reaction to acute illness
- (c) is present in very high concentration in the serum in cirrhosis
- (d) contains some immunoglobulins
- (e) contains haptoglobin.

227 In acute inflammation
- (a) most acute phase reactants are synthesized in the liver
- (b) C-reactive protein acts as an activator of other inflammatory pathways
- (c) the inflammatory response is increased by the presence of α_1-antitrypsin
- (d) measurement of acute phase reactants is useful in determining the cause of the inflammation
- (e) C-reactive protein estimation is less useful than in chronic inflammation.

228 The following changes in the serum protein electrophoretic
     pattern are compatible with a diagnosis of nephrotic syndrome:
     (a) low albumin as the sole abnormality
     (b) low α_1-globulins
     (c) low γ-globulins
     (d) very high β-globulins
     (e) raised γ-globulins.

229 α_1-antitrypsin deficiency
     (a) is usually associated with a reduced density of the α_1-
          globulin band on electrophoresis
     (b) may present in childhood with cirrhosis of the liver
     (c) is a recognized complication of treatment with oral
          contraceptives
     (d) is associated with a subnormal proteolytic action in
          inflammation
     (e) may present in young adults as emphysema.

230 IgM
     (a) can be synthesized by the fetus
     (b) is synthesized as the primary response to particulate antigens
     (c) consists of four immunoglobulin subunits
     (d) deficiency is commonly associated with septicaemia
     (e) concentration reaches adult levels in the plasma by the age
          of nine months.

231 Consequences of the process of complement activation include
     (a) lysis of organisms
     (b) reduction in vascular permeability
     (c) attraction of phagocytes
     (d) opsonization of foreign cells
     (e) formation of antigen-antibody complexes.

232 The C_3 component of complement
     (a) is an α_1-globulin
     (b) is the first component of complement to be activated in the
          classical pathway
     (c) is in low concentration in the plasma in both post-strepto-
          coccal and mesangiocapillary glomerulonephritis
     (d) rises in concentration in the plasma during recovery from
          post-streptococcal glomerulonephritis
     (e) is deficient in hereditary angioneurotic oedema.

233   In an immunoglobulin molecule
    (a)   the immunoglobulin class is determined by the structure of
        the light chains
    (b)   both heavy and light chains are present at the antigen-
        combining sites
    (c)   the structure of the polypeptide chains is variable at the
        antigen-combining sites
    (d)   one light chain is of κ and the other of λ type
    (e)   the heavy chains only are responsible for the ability of the
        molecule to fix complement.

234   The Svedberg coefficient of an immunoglobulin is
    (a)   determined largely by the amino acid composition of the
        light chains
    (b)   19S for IgM
    (c)   related to the density of the molecule
    (d)   7S for IgG
    (e)   4.5S for IgA.

235.   The main functions of the immunoglobulins are as follows:
    (a)   IgG — protection of tissue spaces
    (b)   IgA — protection of body surfaces
    (c)   IgM — protection of the blood stream
    (d)   IgE — neutralization of toxins
    (e)   IgD — immediate hypersensitivity reactions mediated by
        tissue-bound antibodies.

236   Deficiency of
    (a)   immunoglobulins is more often primary than secondary to
        other disease
    (b)   IgG is a recognized complication of prematurity
    (c)   IgA is a characteristic feature of Crohn's disease
    (d)   immunoglobulins may be genetically determined
    (e)   immunoglobulins is a recognized feature of leukaemia.

237   Paraproteinaemia
    (a)   is due to the production of protein different in structure
        from that of normal immunoglobulin
    (b)   is often due to a B cell malignancy
    (c)   is a constant feature of myeloma
    (d)   may be transient
    (e)   is not a feature of soft tissue plasmacytoma unless there is
        bone marrow involvement.

238   Recognized clinical manifestations of myelomatosis include
    (a)   an increasing incidence after the age of 50
    (b)   bone pain
    (c)   anaemia
    (d)   Raynaud's phenomenon
    (e)   lymphadenopathy.

239   In myelomatosis
      (a) renal failure and amyloidosis are related in their aetiology
      (b) light chains of either κ or λ type are found in the urine of about 70 per cent of patients
      (c) the most common paraprotein is IgA
      (d) bone marrow examination is an essential step in the diagnosis
      (e) the presence of Bence Jones protein in the plasma suggests that renal failure is present.

240   Recognized laboratory findings in myelomatosis include
      (a) hypercalcaemia
      (b) raised serum alkaline phosphatase level
      (c) raised ESR
      (d) immune paresis
      (e) low plasma sodium concentration.

241   Recognized features of Waldenström's macroglobulinaemia include
      (a) a greater incidence in females than in males
      (b) intestinal lymphomatous lesions with malabsorption
      (c) Bence Jones proteinuria
      (d) impairment of vision
      (e) raised serum concentration of IgA.

242   Cryoglobulinaemia
      (a) does not occur in Waldenström's macroglobulinaemia
      (b) should not be diagnosed if no paraprotein is found in the serum
      (c) may be associated with immune complex disease
      (d) can be confidently diagnosed as 'essential' if the patient is symptom free
      (e) is likely to be missed unless the blood sample is cooled rapidly after collection.

243   Recognized causes of the nephrotic syndrome include
      (a) 'minimal change' glomerulonephritis
      (b) diabetes mellitus
      (c) amyloidosis
      (d) pyelonephritis
      (e) systemic lupus erythematosus.

244   Typical laboratory findings in a severe case of the nephrotic syndrome include
      (a) hypercalcaemia
      (b) hypoalbuminaemia
      (c) hypercholesterolaemia
      (d) Bence Jones proteinuria
      (e) hypertriglyceridaemia.

245   In the nephrotic syndrome
      (a)   proteinuria ranges up to 50 g per day
      (b)   a ratio of IgG to transferrin clearance of more than 0.2
            implies a good prognosis
      (c)   return of the serum protein concentrations to normal is not
            necessarily a favourable prognostic feature
      (d)   a history of residence abroad may give a clue to the cause
      (e)   turbidity of the plasma is a feature of mild cases.

246   The Albustix test for urinary protein
      (a)   is unreliable if the urine is infected
      (b)   depends on the formation of a protein-indicator complex
      (c)   may be falsely positive if acid is added to the urine as a
            preservative
      (d)   produces a red or orange-red colour if protein is present
      (e)   may be falsely negative if the urine is very dilute.

247   A false positive salicylsulphonic acid test for protein may be due
      to
      (a)   the presence of phosphates
      (b)   contamination of the container with antiseptic
      (c)   a high concentration of urate
      (d)   a recent intravenous pyelogram
      (e)   the administration of tolbutamide.

Chapter XV
Plasma Enzymes in Diagnosis

248 The accurate assessment of tissue damage by estimation of the activity of enzymes in plasma is influenced by the fact that
(a) the estimations must be carried out at precisely $37°C$
(b) the rate at which damage is occurring is at least as important as its extent
(c) enzymes with identical actions liberated from different tissues can sometimes be distinguished by physical or chemical means
(d) the half-lives of most enzymes in the circulation are very much the same
(e) plasma enzyme levels may fall following the total destruction of the affected cells.

249 Haemolysis is an important cause of raised levels of
(a) aspartate transaminase
(b) lactate dehydrogenase
(c) alanine transaminase
(d) alkaline phosphatase
(e) total acid phosphatase.

250 The diagnostic significance of the finding of an elevated plasma level of an enzyme
(a) is low if the patient is in circulatory failure
(b) is unlikely to be increased if the test is repeated after a day or two
(c) is not impaired by haemolysis of the specimen if the enzyme is not present in red cells
(d) can be increased by the estimation of different molecular forms of the enzyme
(e) can be increased by estimation of other enzymes.

251 Non-specific elevation of plasma enzyme levels can occur
(a) after physical exercise
(b) in the neonatal period
(c) in pregnancy
(d) after intravenous injection of suxamethonium
(e) in epileptics.

252 Physiological processes and the abbrevations for the appropriate enzymes are correctly paired below:
(a) transfer of an amino group from glutamate to oxaloacetate — GGT
(b) hydrolysis of phosphates — ALP and ACP
(c) transfer of an amino group from glutamate to pyruvate — ALT
(d) breakdown of dietary starch to maltose — AMS
(e) reversible interconversion of lactate and pyruvate — LD.

253 Conditions in which the plasma level of aspartate transaminase
is relatively very much higher than that of alanine transaminase
include
(a) circulatory failure
(b) viral hepatitis
(c) infectious mononucleosis
(d) extensive trauma
(e) hepatic cirrhosis.

254 Of the five isoenzymes of lactate dehydrogenase
(a) LD_5 is the most abundant form in the liver
(b) LD_1 is the fastest moving fraction on electrophoresis
(c) LD_1 is active against hydroxybutyrate
(d) LD_3 is produced by some malignant tumours
(e) LD_5 levels are typically raised in plasma in active renal disease.

255 Creatine kinase
(a) levels in the plasma are consistently raised in patients with
neurogenic muscular atrophy
(b) plasma levels are a useful screening test for carcinoma of the
lung, especially if a rise in the BB fraction can be demonstrated
(c) isoenzyme of the MB type is detectable in the plasma after
myocardial infarction
(d) levels in the plasma are moderately raised in hypothyroidism
(e) levels in the plasma usually start to rise earlier than those of
any other enzyme after myocardial infarction.

256 A raised plasma total amylase level
(a) is useful in the differential diagnosis of chronic abdominal
pain
(b) may be found as a result of the administration of morphine
(c) is a recognized finding in severe diabetic ketoacidosis
(d) is a recognized feature of mumps
(e) without a raised urinary level is diagnostic of renal failure.

257 The finding of a raised plasma level of
(a) alkaline phosphatase together with a raised level of γ-glutamyl
transferase occurs in cholestatic jaundice of pregnancy
(b) heat-stable alkaline phosphatase is of no clinical significance
in pregnancy
(c) alkaline phosphatase together with a raised level of total acid
phosphatase is compatible with a diagnosis of Paget's disease
(d) heat-stable alkaline phosphatase in a male is compatible with
a diagnosis of bronchial carcinoma
(e) alkaline phosphatase is to be expected at puberty.

258 Typically the plasma level of acid phosphatase
(a) of the tartrate-stable type is used as a marker for prostatic
carcinoma
(b) is raised following rectal examination and the estimation
should be repeated after 24 hours
(c) is raised in Gaucher's disease
(d) is below normal in cretinism
(e) is moderately raised in muscle diseases.

259 The following findings in plasma are usually compatible with a
      myocardial infarction 24-48 hours previously:
  (a) raised aspartate transaminase level
  (b) raised creatine kinase level
  (c) slightly raised alanine transaminase level
  (d) undetectable MB isoenzyme of creatine kinase
  (e) normal hydroxybutyrate dehydrogenase level.

260 Following a myocardial infarction
  (a) the plasma hydroxybutrate dehydrogenase level may well be
        raised after 10 days
  (b) the plasma enzyme levels may remain normal
  (c) a secondary rise in plasma hydroxybutyrate dehydrogenase
        level is compatible with a diagnosis of congestive heart failure
  (d) the extent of the rise in plasma aspartate transaminase is an
        accurate measure of the size of the infarct
  (e) estimation of creatine kinase isoenzymes is hardly ever
        necessary for diagnosis.

261 In the Duchenne type of muscular dystrophy
  (a) the plasma creatine kinase level rises progressively as the
        disease advances
  (b) the plasma transaminase levels are typically normal
  (c) the plasma creatine kinase level is at its highest after a
        prolonged period of rest
  (d) in neonates, plasma levels of creatine kinase are usually
        within the normal adult range
  (e) carriers typically show a moderate rise in plasma creatine
        kinase levels.

262 Elevated levels of plasma cholinesterase (pseudo-cholinesterase)
      are typically found in
  (a) hepatic cirrhosis
  (b) nephrotic syndrome
  (c) myocardial infarction
  (d) organophosphate poisoning
  (e) fluoride poisoning.

263 In patients with inherited suxamethonium sensitivity
  (a) prolonged apnoea may follow administration of the muscle
        relaxant
  (b) who are homozygous, cholinesterase is absent from the
        plasma
  (c) the abnormal cholinesterase is more completely inhibited by
        dibucaine than is the normal enzyme
  (d) marked sensitivity is generally only found in homozygotes
  (e) examination of other members of the family is essential.

Chapter XVI
Inborn Errors of Metabolism

264 Inherited biochemical abnormalities
(a) are usually due to defective synthesis of a single peptide
(b) are always life-threatening unless treated
(c) are less serious if the metabolic pathway affected is controlled by feedback
(d) can cause accumulation of a metabolite of the substrate acted upon by an affected enzyme
(e) may become clinically manifest only after the administration of a drug.

265 The following clinical findings, without obvious cause in children, are suggestive of an inborn error of metabolism:
(a) enlargement of the kidneys
(b) virilism
(c) hypoglycaemia
(d) failure to thrive
(e) renal calculi.

266 In order to prevent irreversible clinical consequences or death, it is important to make an early diagnosis of
(a) Hartnup disease
(b) alkaptonuria
(c) phenylketonuria
(d) renal glycosuria
(e) maple syrup urine disease.

267 A father is heterozygous for an abnormal autosomal gene and has a clinically manifest disorder in consequence; the mother is normal. It is statistically likely that
(a) all their children will carry the abnormal gene
(b) about a quarter of their children will be heterozygous
(c) about half their chidren will suffer from the disorder
(d) the disorder is unlikely to occur in their grandchildren
(e) one of the father's parents must have been homozygous for the abnormal gene.

268 In a disorder characterized by X-linked recessive inheritance
(a) none of the sons of an affected father and a genetically normal mother will have the disorder
(b) all the sons of a carrier mother will be affected
(c) half the daughters of an affected father will have affected sons
(d) females are never affected
(e) the abnormal gene is usually carried on both female X chromosomes.

269 Aminoaciduria
  (a) due to severe hepatic disease is usually associated with
       increased renal excretion of phosphate
  (b) of specific type is almost always due to a genetically
       determined defect of renal tubular absorption
  (c) of non-specific type is more often associated with high than
       with low plasma levels of amino acids
  (d) in the Fanconi syndrome is usually due to an acquired renal
       lesion
  (e) does not occur if proximal renal tubular reabsorptive
       capacity is normal.

270 The amino acids excreted in excess in the urine in cystinuria
     include
  (a) ornithine
  (b) arginine
  (c) leucine
  (d) glycine
  (e) proline.

271 In cystinuria
  (a) the most important clinical manifestation is renal calculus
       formation
  (b) the intestinal absorption of cystine is increased
  (c) a high fluid intake should be maintained
  (d) renal tubular damage may result from the intracellular
       accumulation of cystine
  (e) the urine should be acidified to increase the solubility of
       cystine.

272 Characteristic features of Hartnup disease include
  (a) increased urinary excretion of tryptophan
  (b) cerebellar ataxia
  (c) a response to treatment with nicotinamide
  (d) non-specific aminoaciduria
  (e) excessive excretion of indole compounds in the urine.

273 Recognized features of phenylketonuria include
  (a) a placid disposition
  (b) vomiting in the first few weeks of life
  (c) pigmentation of the skin
  (d) generalized eczema
  (e) mental retardation by the age of 4-6 months.

274 In phenylketonuria
  (a) the main metabolic abnormality is a deficiency of tyrosinase
  (b) phenylpyruvic acid is excreted in excess in the urine
  (c) phenylalanine accumulates in the blood
  (d) tyrosine levels in the blood are high
  (e) permanent cerebral damage does not occur until after the
       Phenistix test becomes positive.

275   The following statements are correct:
   (a) Estimation of blood phenylalanine is not suitable for routine
        screening for phenylketonuria.
   (b) Phenylketonuria is occasionally caused by an abnormality in
        synthesis of tetrahydrobiopterin.
   (c) Persistent hyperphenylalaninaemia is unequivocal evidence of
        phenylketonuria.
   (d) All the babies of untreated phenylketonuric mothers are at
        risk of developing mental retardation.
   (e) Both phenylalanine and tyrosine must be excluded from the
        diet if the effects of phenylketonuria are to be prevented.

276   Recognized features of alkaptonuria include
   (a) chronic arthritis
   (b) glycosuria
   (c) darkening of the ears
   (d) a normal expectation of life
   (e) the passage of black urine.

277   A genetically determined primary defect of amino acid
      metabolism is responsible for the presence of the following
      substances in the urine in the diseases named:
   (a) valine in maple syrup urine disease
   (b) imidazole pyruvic acid in histidinaemia
   (c) tryptophan in Wilson's disease
   (d) tyrosine in Hartnup disease
   (e) homogentisic acid in familial iminoglycinuria.

278   In Wilson's disease
   (a) blindness frequently occurs as a result of copper deposition
        in the cornea
   (b) degeneration of the pyramidal tracts is a characteristic
        feature
   (c) hepatic cirrhosis is a recognized feature
   (d) liver biopsy may be needed for diagnosis
   (e) D-penicillamine is a recommended treatment.

279   The following drugs are known to cause haemolysis in patients
      with glucose-6-phosphate dehydrogenase deficiency:
   (a) barbiturates
   (b) primaquine
   (c) halothane
   (d) sulphonamides
   (e) vitamin K analogues.

280   The following disorders are inherited as autosomal recessive
      traits:
   (a) malignant hyperpyrexia
   (b) cystinosis
   (c) Hartnup disease
   (d) phenylketonuria
   (e) renal glycosuria.

Chapter XVII
Purine and Urate Metabolism

281   In the synthesis of purines
     (a) the rate-limiting step is the conversion of phosphoribosyl pyrophosphate to phosphoribosylamine
     (b) amino groups are incorporated from glutamine and glycine
     (c) the final stage is the addition of ribose phosphate
     (d) nucleic acids are formed in the intermediate stages
     (e) the rate-limiting step is subject to feedback inhibition from increased levels of purine nucleotides.

282   The formation of urate
     (a) from adenine is via the formation of xanthine
     (b) from guanine is via the formation of hypoxanthine
     (c) from purines depends on xanthine oxidase activity
     (d) from xanthine is via hypoxanthine
     (e) is the last stage of purine breakdown in most mammals.

283   The following statements about urate excretion are correct:
     (a) Urinary excretion is increased by probenecid.
     (b) About half of the urate filtered at the glomerulus is reabsorbed in the tubule.
     (c) Active tubular secretion of urate occurs.
     (d) Thiazide diuretics inhibit renal excretion.
     (e) Renal excretion is inhibited by lactic acid.

284   The precipitation of urate
     (a) in tissues is probably enhanced by local tissue acidosis
     (b) in acute gouty arthritis is more dependent on the plasma urate level than on local factors
     (c) in the subcutaneous tissue causes severe pain
     (d) in the kidney can cause renal failure
     (e) in tissues may be caused by trauma.

285   Hyperuricaemia
     (a) is commoner in men than women
     (b) can be inherited as a sex-linked recessive trait
     (c) has a recognized association with hypercalcaemia
     (d) is commoner after the menopause than before
     (e) is a recognized complication of alcoholism.

286 In primary hyperuricaemia
- (a) there is probably a failure of feedback inhibition of the rate-limiting step in purine synthesis
- (b) renal clearance of urate is increased unless renal failure is present
- (c) the most effective therapeutic measure is reduction of purine intake
- (d) salicylates in low dosage are a useful therapeutic measure
- (e) allopurinol can be used to inhibit the oxidation of xanthine and hypoxanthine.

287 Characteristic features of the Lesch—Nyhan syndrome include
- (a) failure of conversion of xanthine to urate
- (b) mental deficiency
- (c) self-mutilation
- (d) aggressive behaviour
- (e) spastic paraplegia.

288 Recognized causes of hyperuricaemia include
- (a) leukaemia
- (b) glucose-6-phosphatase deficiency
- (c) chronic starvation
- (d) psoriasis
- (e) xanthinuria.

289 In renal failure
- (a) with a plasma urea of 50 mmol/litre, a plasma urate of 0.6 mmol/litre suggests that hyperuricaemia is the cause
- (b) clinical gout is rarely associated with secondary hyperuricaemia
- (c) the rise of plasma urate is proportionally greater than that of urea
- (d) the rise in plasma urate stimulates the deposition of calcium pyrophosphate in joint cavities
- (e) developing acutely in a patient being treated by radiotherapy, tubular blockage by uric acid is a possible cause.

Chapter XVIII
Iron Metabolism

290 The following statements are correct:
   (a) Up to 25 per cent of the body iron is in the ferric state.
   (b) Iron overload is evident when stainable iron is demonstrable in the reticulo-endothelial cells in the bone marrow.
   (c) Less than 1 per cent of the body iron is circulating, bound to protein, in the plasma.
   (d) Iron in the reduced state is present in 'reduced' haemoglobin but not in oxyhaemoglobin.
   (e) About 70 per cent of the body iron is in haemoglobin.

291 The average amount of iron lost daily from the body by
   (a) a normal man is about 18 μmol (1 mg)
   (b) an adolescent boy is as high as that lost by a menstruating woman
   (c) a pregnant woman is about 45 μmol (2.5 mg)
   (d) a male blood donor giving a pint of blood three times a year is about 36 μmol (2 mg)
   (e) a normal menstruating woman is about 27 μmol (1.5 mg).

292 Plasma iron concentration
   (a) is higher in men than in women
   (b) is higher in the evening than in the morning
   (c) falls in the early weeks of pregnancy
   (d) can vary, apparently at random, as much as threefold from day to day
   (e) rises in women who start taking some oral contraceptives.

293 Plasma iron concentration is typically higher than normal in
   (a) rheumatoid arthritis
   (b) folate deficiency
   (c) acute haemolytic episodes
   (d) hypochromic microcytic anaemia
   (e) acute liver disease.

294 Iron stores in the bone marrow are usually increased in
   (a) chronic infection
   (b) thalassaemia
   (c) chronic haemolytic anaemia
   (d) idiopathic haemochromatosis
   (e) bone marrow hypoplasia.

295   The total iron-binding capacity
   (a)   is used as an indirect measure of the plasma transferrin concentration
   (b)   is normally about six times the plasma iron concentration
   (c)   should be measured only if the plasma iron concentration is normal
   (d)   rises in women on some oral contraceptives
   (e)   is less labile than the plasma iron concentration.

296   Similar changes (rise or fall) in the total iron-binding capacity and the plasma iron concentration typically occur in
   (a)   iron-deficiency anaemia
   (b)   malignancy
   (c)   iron overload
   (d)   late pregnancy
   (e)   nephrotic syndrome.

297   The administration of iron
   (a)   by a parenteral route is particularly indicated in chronic renal disease
   (b)   by the oral route cannot cause iron overload if the patient is not anaemic
   (c)   by the oral route is contraindicated in chronic haemolytic anaemia
   (d)   by a parenteral route leads to an increased renal excretion of iron
   (e)   is clearly indicated if the plasma iron concentration is below normal.

298   Iron deposition
   (a)   in excess in the bonemarrow is compatible with a reduction in haemoglobin iron
   (b)   as a result of multiple blood transfusions is characteristically associated with tissue damage
   (c)   in the liver as a result of excessive iron intake is exclusively in the parenchymal cells
   (d)   in association with tissue damage is called haemochromatosis
   (e)   may result from a genetically determined excess of transferrin.

299   Recognized features of haemochromatosis include
   (a)   diabetes mellitus
   (b)   hepatocellular carcinoma
   (c)   osteoporosis
   (d)   hypogonadism
   (e)   cardiac failure.

300   The following statements about idiopathic haemochromatosis
      are correct:
      (a) Plasma ferritin levels may be normal.
      (b) The skin pigmentation is due to the colour of deposited iron.
      (c) It should not be diagnosed unless increased intestinal absorp-
           tion of iron can be demonstrated.
      (d) Removal of the excess iron stores will usually cause iron
           absorption to return to normal.
      (e) Examination of liver biopsy material easily distinguishes this
           condition from alcoholic cirrhosis.

301   Recognized features of the syndrome of dietary iron overload
      described in the black population of Southern Africa include
      (a) a genetically determined increased absorption of ingested
           iron
      (b) a poor response to chelating agents
      (c) deposition of iron in excess in the bone marrow
      (d) scurvy
      (e) hepatic cirrhosis.

Chapter XIX
The Porphyrias

302 In the synthesis of haem
   (a) the rate-limiting step is the condensation of glycine and
       succinate to form 5-aminolaevulinate (ALA)
   (b) porphobilinogen (PBG) is formed from two molecules of
       ALA
   (c) the formation of coproporphyrinogen precedes that of
       uroporphyrinogen
   (d) iron is incorporated into protoporphyrin
   (e) the rate-limiting step is catalysed by ALA-synthase.

303 The following substances fluoresce in ultraviolet light:
   (a) 5-aminolaevulinate
   (b) porphobilinogen
   (c) uroporphyrinogen III
   (d) protoporphyrin III
   (e) coproporphyrin III.

304 Darkening on standing of a specimen of urine could be due to the
     presence of
   (a) coproporphyrinogen III
   (b) porphobilinogen
   (c) protoporphyrin
   (d) uroporphyrinogen I
   (e) uroporphyrinogen III.

305 Recognized manifestations of the inherited porphyrias include
   (a) photosensitivity of the skin
   (b) ulcerative lesions of the upper gastro-intestinal tract
   (c) peripheral neuritis
   (d) colicky abdominal pain
   (e) quadriplegia.

306 In the latent phase of
   (a) the hepatic porphyrias recurrent mild abdominal pain is a
       typical feature
   (b) porphyria variegata photosensitivity can be expected
   (c) acute intermittent porphyria porphyrins are usually found in
       the faeces
   (d) hereditary coproporphyria an increase in urinary
       porphobilinogen can be detected
   (e) acute intermittent porphyria skin lesions do not occur.

307   ALA synthase activity is increased
      (a) in all the hepatic porphyrias
      (b) in congenital erythropoietic porphyria
      (c) by increased levels of haem
      (d) by the administration of barbiturates
      (e) by the administration of sulphonamides.

308   The following disorders are inherited as autosomal dominant
      traits:
      (a) acute intermittent porphyria
      (b) hereditary coproporphyria
      (c) porphyria variegata
      (d) congenital erythropoietic porphyria
      (e) erythrohepatic protoporphyria.

309   Recognized features of acute attacks of acute intermittent
      porphyria include
      (a) severe blistering of the skin
      (b) an increase in urinary ALA and PBG
      (c) an onset after puberty
      (d) death from respiratory paralysis
      (e) increased urinary porphyrin excretion.

310   Screening tests
      (a) on urine for acute intermittent porphyria are unreliable in
           the latent phase
      (b) in adults for faecal porphyrins can, if negative, reliably
           exclude porphyria variegata
      (c) in children for acute intermittent porphyria should include
           estimation of uroporphyrinogen-1-synthase in erythrocytes
      (d) must be carried out on relations of any known porphyric
      (e) for the inherited porphyrias may be positive in patients with
           chronic haemorrhage from haemorrhoids.

311   Typical features of porphyria cutanea tarda include
      (a) excessive urinary excretion of uroporphyrin 1
      (b) severe photosensitivity
      (c) hirsutism
      (d) severe anaemia
      (e) hyperpigmentation.

Chapter XX
Vitamins

312   The fat-soluble vitamins include vitamin
    (a)   D
    (b) B_{12}
    (c)   A
    (d) B_1
    (e)   K

313   Vitamin A
    (a)   is formed by the hydrolysis of a substance found in the green and yellow parts of plants
    (b)   is not stored in significant amounts in the human body
    (c)   is rapidly destroyed by ultraviolet light
    (d)   given in large doses for long periods causes desquamation and pigmentation of the skin
    (e)   is essential for normal collagen synthesis.

314   Deficiency of vitamin A
    (a)   is associated with poor scotopic vision
    (b)   is unlikely to occur in children whose diet contains plenty of carotene
    (c)   is an important cause of blindness in underdeveloped countries
    (d)   is the cause of some of the typical manifestations of intestinal malabsorption
    (e)   is a recognized cause of squamous carcinoma of the skin.

315   Foods which are particularly rich in thiamine include
    (a)   citrus fruits
    (b)   wheat germ
    (c)   oatmeal
    (d)   polished rice
    (e)   yeast.

316   Recognized consequences of thiamine deficiency include
    (a)   polyneuropathy
    (b)   cheilosis
    (c)   cardiac failure
    (d)   reduced level of pyruvate in the blood
    (e)   reduced erythrocyte transketolase activity.

317 The following statements are correct:
  (a) Dietary deficiency of vitamin K does not occur.
  (b) Bitot's spots are a feature of severe xerosis conjunctivae.
  (c) Pantothenate deficiency causes the tongue to become
       magenta coloured.
  (d) The administration of isoniazid can produce the clinical
       picture of riboflavin deficiency.
  (e) Beriberi can be aggravated by a low carbohydrate diet.

318 Characteristic features of pellagra include
  (a) dementia
  (b) hypochromic microcytic anaemia
  (c) depression
  (d) diarrhoea
  (e) pigmentation of the skin.

319 Nicotinic acid
  (a) can be converted in the body to nicotinamide
  (b) is absorbed poorly from the intestine in Hartnup disease
  (c) is probably synthesized from tryptophan in less than normal
       amounts in the carcinoid syndrome
  (d) is a co-enzyme for the transaminases
  (e) requires pyridoxal phosphate for its normal synthesis from
       tryptophan.

320 Folate
  (a) in the form of tetrahydrofolate is necessary for the synthesis
       of nucleic acids
  (b) antagonists can cause subacute combined degeneration of
       the spinal cord
  (c) deficiency is a recognized complication of pregnancy
  (d) does not improve the megaloblastic anaemia of vitamin B_{12}
       deficiency
  (e) and vitamin B_{12} have similar co-enzyme activity.

321 Scurvy
  (a) is a common complication of intestinal malabsorption
  (b) is more likely to occur in breast-fed than in bottle-fed infants
  (c) occurs if ascorbate is oxidized to dehydroascorbate by heat
  (d) is most commonly seen in old men living alone
  (e) is probably best diagnosed in the laboratory by plasma
       ascorbate assay.

322 Recognized manifestations of ascorbate deficiency include
  (a) anaemia in the absence of blood loss
  (b) poor healing of fractures
  (c) permanent joint deformities
  (d) epistaxes
  (e) bone pain in infancy.

Chapter XXI
Pregnancy and Oral Contraceptive Therapy

323   Analysis of amniotic fluid after 28 weeks gestation is of recognized value in the diagnosis or prediction of
   (a) fetoplacental impairment
   (b) fetomaternal blood group incompatibility
   (c) fetal neural tube defects
   (d) respiratory distress syndrome
   (e) threatened abortion.

324   In a normal pregnancy
   (a) the developing placenta secretes progesterone until about the 13th week
   (b) oestriol excretion in the urine is difficult to measure until after the 28th week
   (c) the plasma oestriol concentration is generally accepted to be the most reliable predictor of intact fetoplacental function
   (d) chorionic gonadotrophin controls placental secretion of oestriol and progesterone
   (e) fetoplacental function can be measured by radio-immuno-assay of human placental lactogen.

325   Pulmonary surfactant
   (a) is a polypeptide
   (b) is synthesized from about 33 weeks gestation onwards
   (c) formation can be inferred from the lecithin-sphingomyelin ratio in amniotic fluid
   (d) contains palmitic acid
   (e) acts by increasing the surface tension in the pulmonary alveoli.

326   α-fetoprotein
   (a) is normally present in high concentration in fetal blood at 16—18 weeks
   (b) in low concentration in maternal plasma reliably excludes fetal malformation
   (c) in high concentration in amniotic fluid is a typical finding in anencephaly
   (d) in high concentration in amniotic fluid is a recognized finding in multiple pregnancy
   (e) is a lipoprotein.

327   Recognized effects of pregnancy include
   (a) glycosuria
   (b) a raised glomerular filtration rate
   (c) a raised plasma concentration of free thyroxine
   (d) a raised plasma alkaline phosphatase
   (e) a raised plasma concentration of free cortisol.

328   Amniotic fluid
   (a) sampling by amniocentesis carries no risk to the fetus if
        performed by an expert
   (b) acetylcholinesterase may rise if fetal malformation is present
   (c) is probably derived from both maternal and fetal sources
   (d) bilirubin levels normally increase during the second half of
        pregnancy
   (e) sphingomyelin levels remain constant in late pregnancy.

329   Patients taking oral contraceptives
   (a) rarely develop cholestatic jaundice
   (b) have raised plasma gonadotrophin levels
   (c) usually have a slightly raised plasma albumin
   (d) typically have increased plasma thyroxine-binding globulin
   (e) may develop renal glycosuria.

Chapter XXII
Biochemical Effects of Tumours

330　APUD cells
  (a)　are probably all mesodermal in origin
  (b)　are found in specialized nerve tissue only
  (c)　can remove carboxyl groups from some amino acids
  (d)　can secrete amines and peptide hormones
  (e)　in the bronchial tree are sometimes non-secretory.

331　The following substances are catecholamines:
  (a)　dihydroxyphenylalanine
  (b)　adrenaline
  (c)　dihydroxyphenylethylamine
F (d)　tyrosine
  (e)　norepinephrine.

332　Noradrenaline
  (a)　is almost exclusively a product of the adrenal medulla
T (b)　is broken down to 4-hydroxy 3-methoxy-mandelic acid
T (c)　produces generalized vasoconstriction
  (d)　increases the rate of glycogenolysis
T (e)　is derived directly from dopamine.

333　Recognized features of phaeochromocytoma include
  (a)　glycosuria
  (b)　sustained hypertension
  (c)　facial pallor
  (d)　facial flushing
F (e)　a marked tendency to become malignant.

334　Neuroblastoma
T (a)　occurs in a younger age group than does phaeochromo-
      cytoma
T (b)　is very malignant
  (c)　is found more often in the adrenal medulla than in extra-
      adrenal tissue
  (d)　is associated with only slightly raised secretion of catecho-
      lamines
  (e)　arises in the same type of cells as does phaeochromocytoma.

335 HMMA (VMA) excretion

T   (a) more than twice the upper limit of normal is diagnostic of a
          catecholamine-secreting tumour

T   (b) may be slightly raised in cases of essential hypertension

     (c) persistently within the normal range is incompatible with a
          diagnosis of phaeochromocytoma

     (d) should not be measured until plasma catecholamines have
          been shown to be high

T   (e) in a case of phaeochromocytoma is more likely to be raised
          during and after a paroxysm of hypertension.

336 APUD argentaffin cells

     (a) are most commonly found in the ileum and the appendix

     (b) are the only cells which contain aromatic amino acid
          decarboxylase

     (c) synthesize serotonin from tryptophan via 5-hydroxytrypto-
          phan

     (d) may secrete a peptide in addition to a biologically active
          amine

     (e) contain monoamine oxidases which oxidize 5-hydroxy-
          indole acetic acid.

337 The clinical features of the carcinoid syndrome

     (a) can be produced by a benign tumour of the ileum

     (b) include right-sided cardiac lesions

     (c) are largely attributable to an excess of circulating 5-hydroxy-
          tryptamine

     (d) include bronchospasm

     (e) may include pellagra due to tryptophan deficiency.

338 The Zollinger—Ellison syndrome

     (a) is usually due to a single adenoma of the G cells of the
          pancreatic islets

     (b) can be diagnosed by finding a very low pH of gastric juice in
          association with a high plasma gastrin

     (c) may be associated with a parathyroid adenoma

     (d) may be associated with clinically significant inhibition of
          lipase

     (e) often presents with a bullous rash known as necrolytic
          migratory erythema.

339 The manifestations of a tumour of the A cells of the pancreatic
     islets include

     (a) thrombo-embolism

     (b) profuse watery diarrhoea

     (c) impaired glucose tolerance

     (d) increased urinary excretion of total 5-hydroxyindoles

     (e) psychiatric disturbance.

340 In multiple endocrine adenopathy II (MEA II) the following tumours typically secrete inappropriate amounts of hormones:
(a) thyroid adenoma
(b) adrenal cortical adenoma
(c) medullary carcinoma of the thyroid
(d) phaeochromocytoma
(e) parathyroid adenoma.

341 The secretion of hormones by a bronchial carcinoma
(a) is, by definition, ectopic
(b) may result in high plasma α-fetoprotein levels
(c) is always inappropriate
(d) may, possibly, be due to malignancy of pulmonary APUD cells
(e) causes hypercalcaemia more often than hypoglycaemia.

342 Inappropriate antidiuretic hormone secretion typically causes a reduction of
(a) plasma sodium concentration
(b) urinary sodium concentration
(c) plasma osmolality
(d) arterial blood pressure
(e) aldosterone secretion.

343 The syndrome of inappropriate ACTH secretion
(a) is most often due to a thymic tumour
(b) often presents clinically with Cushingoid features
(c) is associated with an increased secretion of aldosterone
(d) is characterized by alkalosis
(e) is best treated with potassium replacement alone.

344 The following statements are correct:
(a) The association of hypernephroma and polycythaemia is probably due to ectopic hormone production.
(b) The commonest tumour to secrete a substance that reacts like insulin in immunoassays is a large retroperitoneal fibro-sarcoma.
(c) Gynaecomastia is a recognized complication of primary hepatoma.
(d) In carcinoid syndrome due to bronchial carcinoma, the urinary excretion of 5-HT is out of proportion to that of 5-HIAA.
(e) The presence of carcino-embryonic antigen in the serum is reliable evidence of colonic carcinoma.

Chapter XXIII
The Cerebrospinal Fluid

345 Biochemical investigation of the CSF
   (a) should precede bacteriological examination
   (b) is of no value if the fluid is very cloudy
   (c) should always be accompanied by the appropriate chemical
        tests on plasma
   (d) is not indicated if the fluid is xanthochromic
   (e) is not indicated if the fluid is uniformly blood-stained.

346 A very high protein concentration in the CSF together with a
     xanthochromic appearance is characteristic of
   (a) encephalitis
   (b) purulent meningitis
   (c) polyneuritis
   (d) blockage of the spinal canal
   (e) a cerebral tumour near the surface of the brain.

347 Characteristic findings in the CSF in multiple sclerosis include
   (a) xanthochromia
   (b) oligoclonal bands on electrophoresis
   (c) a low glucose concentration
   (d) an albumin concentration which is lower than expected from
        the plasma concentration of albumin
   (e) a tendency to clot.

348 The following statements about the CSF are correct:
   (a) Oligoclonal bands signify cerebral disease only if they are
        found in the CSF *and in the serum*.
   (b) Estimation of glucose concentration is of no value in the
        diagnosis of tuberculous meningitis.
   (c) Intrathecal malignant B cells may cause a local monoclonal
        band.
   (d) Unconjugated hyperbilirubinaemia may cause
        xanthochromia.
   (e) Measurement of CSF total protein is a sensitive test for
        cerebral disease.

Chapter XXIV
Drug Monitoring

349 In assessing the active concentration of a drug in plasma, it is important to remember that:
    (a) Protein binding partially inactivates many drugs.
    (b) Most assays measure the total of the free plus the protein bound drug concentrations.
    (c) A reduction in protein binding will lead to a reduction in the total concentration of a drug.
    (d) There is a linear relationship between albumin concentration and the concentration of protein bound drug.
    (e) If several drugs are present they may compete for the same protein binding sites.

350 In suspected paracetamol poisoning
    (a) plasma paracetamol levels are not relevant because it is a metabolite that is toxic
    (b) diagnosis is important because a specific antidote is available
    (c) the clinical state of the patient at presentation usually indicates whether or not hepatotoxicity is likely to develop
    (d) absorption and distribution can be assumed to be complete two hours after ingestion
    (e) treatment involves increasing the urinary excretion of paracetamol.

351 Estimation of plasma anticonvulsant levels is useful
    (a) to assess compliance
    (b) if toxicity is suspected clinically
    (c) in children
    (d) if the frequency of fits increases
    (e) in pregnant women.

352 In digoxin therapy
    (a) random plasma levels are important in monitoring treatment
    (b) elderly patients often have a low threshold for toxicity
    (c) a given level of digoxin may have increased effect in the presence of hyperkalaemia
    (d) about 20 per cent of digoxin is protein bound
    (e) tissue sensitivity is increased by hypercalcaemia.

353 The following statements about drug overdosage are correct:
    (a) Excretion of most barbiturates is easily increased.
    (b) Iron overdosage most commonly occurs in children.
    (c) It is almost always necessary to measure plasma drug levels.
    (d) Interpretation of plasma lithium assays is complicated by protein abnormalities.
    (e) Many patients attempting suicide take several drugs.

Chapters XXV and XXVI
The Clinician's Contribution; Requesting Tests and Interpreting Results

354 The following statements are correct:
  (a) Plasma drug levels should be estimated at a standard time after the dose.
  (b) Significant hypokalaemia may occur for a few hours after taking a single dose of a diuretic.
  (c) Salicylates may cause the plasma total T_4 concentration to appear falsely high.
  (d) The rise in plasma concentration of tartrate-labile acid phosphatase following rectal examination can last as long as three days.
  (e) Blood sampling during an infusion of lipid will interfere with the plasma sodium estimation, resulting in a spurious hypernatraemia.

355 Prolonged stasis during venepuncture can cause an increased plasma concentration of the following substances:
  (a) calcium
  (b) sodium
  (c) potassium
  (d) immunoglobulins
  (e) thyroxine.

356 If a patient is receiving an intravenous infusion in the right arm blood taken
  (a) from a right arm vein distal to the infusion site can be regarded as chemically representative of the patient's circulating blood
  (b) from a right arm vein proximal to the infusion site will always have concentrations of plasma electrolytes which are obviously incorrect
  (c) from a vein in the left arm can be regarded as representative of the patient's circulating blood
  (d) should in no circumstances be taken via the needle of the infusion set
  (e) from a right arm vein proximal to the infusion site yielding results of plasma sodium 65 mmol/litre and plasma glucose 50 mmol/litre is compatible with the infusion being of dextrose.

357 Errors can be expected in the estimation of the following plasma constituents if the blood is mixed with the substances listed with them
    (a) fluoride : glucose
    (b) sequestrene : potassium
    (c) lithium heparin : sodium
    (d) ethylene-diamine tetracetate : calcium
    (e) sodium oxalate : calcium.

358 Whole blood containing an anticoagulant and left overnight
    (a) will have a falsely high potassium concentration
    (b) will have a falsely low glucose concentration
    (c) can safely be used for chemical analysis if it has been stored in a refrigerator
    (d) will have a falsely high bilirubin concentration
    (e) can be recognized by the red colour of the plasma.

359 The following statements about collection of urine or faeces for chemical study are correct:
    (a) A 24-hour urine collection must include the specimens passed both at the beginning and the end of the 24 hours.
    (b) The commonest cause of an incomplete urine collection is impairment of bladder function.
    (c) Collection of faeces for fat estimation should continue for at least three days.
    (d) A preservative must usually be added to faeces.
    (e) A purgative should be given to constipated patients to ensure complete collection of faeces.

360 The following statements are correct:
    (a) A high plasma potassium concentration may be associated with intracellular depletion.
    (b) A low plasma sodium concentration may occur even when there is an excess of sodium in the body.
    (c) It is unnecessary to measure T_4 and TSH levels in a patient with overt hypothyroidism.
    (d) Plasma urea concentration usually becomes abnormal during the first 12 hours of anuria.
    (e) It is important to perform daily transaminase estimations in a patient with acute hepatitis.

361   The following statements are correct:
   (a)   If a 'normal' range for the concentration of a substance is quoted as the 90 per cent limits, one normal subject out of 40 can be expected to have a level above the upper limit.
   (b)   A plasma urea concentration of 7.5 mmol/litre (45 mg/dl) cannot be regarded as evidence of renal damage at the age of 70.
   (c)   Inter-laboratory variation in plasma enzyme estimations can be eliminated if the internationally accepted methods of estimation are used.
   (d)   A low plasma sodium concentration is more likely to be due to sodium depletion than to overhydration.
   (e)   Out-patients tend to have lower plasma albumin concentrations than do in-patients.

362   Reproducible variations in concentration of some plasma constituents occur
   (a)   in relation to meals
   (b)   throughout the 24 hours
   (c)   from one day to the next
   (d)   over a monthly cycle
   (e)   in relation to posture.

Part Two

Section A

In this section the questions are of the same type as in Part One, i.e. the Independent True/False type. These questions may deal with material from more than one chapter of *Clinical Chemistry in Diagnosis and Treatment*.

363 Reduction of glomerular filtration rate sufficient to cause a raised plasma urea occurs in
    (a) congestive cardiac failure
    (b) obstruction of the urethra
    (c) early nephrotic syndrome
    (d) acute glomerulonephritis
    (e) Addison's disease.

364 Impairment of intrinsic renal function is almost certainly present if an adult patient has
    (a) a plasma urea of 9 mmol/litre (54 mg/dl)
    (b) a plasma creatinine of 300 μmol/litre (3.4 mg/dl)
    (c) a maximum urine osmolality of less than 850 mmol/kg after taking no fluids for 12 hours
    (d) a plasma urate over 0.55 mmol/litre (9 mg/dl)
    (e) proteinuria amounting to 3 g daily.

365 Urinary calculi containing calcium may be the result of
    (a) renal tubular acidosis
    (b) secondary hyperparathyroidism
    (c) vitamin D intoxication
    (d) idiopathic hypercalciuria
    (e) chronic renal infection.

366 Antidiuretic hormone (arginine vasopressin)
    (a) is normally produced in the hypothalamus
    (b) is secreted by the posterior pituitary gland
    (c) exerts its effects through a reduction in the glomerular filtration rate
    (d) ceases to be secreted if the plasma osmotic pressure falls by two per cent
    (e) secretion is inhibited in the recovery phase of acute oliguric renal failure.

367 The following mechanisms play an important part in maintaining
     the blood pH within normal limits:
     (a) conversion of carbonate to bicarbonate through the action
          of the enzyme carbonate dehydratase
     (b) increased pulmonary ventilation in response to a rise in
          blood CO_2 concentration
     (c) buffering of hydrogen ions from carbonic acid by
          erythrocyte haemoglobin
     (d) diffusion of chloride into erythrocytes when CO_2 is taken up
          by the blood
     (e) decreased renal tubular generation of bicarbonate in
          response to a rise in blood CO_2 concentration.

368 The combination of low arterial PO_2 with high arterial PCO_2 is
     characteristic of respiratory failure due to
     (a) pulmonary oedema
     (b) ankylosing spondylitis
     (c) poliomyelitis
     (d) chronic bronchitis
     (e) gross obesity.

369 Pituitary secretion of ACTH (corticotrophin) is increased
     (a) when the subject is exposed to physical stress
     (b) when the subject is exposed to mental stress
     (c) in the evening (10 p.m.--midnight approx)
     (d) when cortisol production is reduced
     (e) in acromegaly.

370 Cushing's syndrome may be due to
     (a) a basophil adenoma of the pituitary
     (b) carcinoma of the bronchus
     (c) adenoma of the adrenal cortex
     (d) excessive secretion of prolactin in the male
     (e) argentaffin tumour of the appendix.

371 The plasma thyroxine concentration is high in
     (a) nephrotic syndrome
     (b) inherited TBG excess
     (c) Hashimoto's disease
     (d) the first month of life
     (e) hypercholesterolaemia.

372 In diabetic ketoacidosis
     (a) the plasma total protein level is typically low
     (b) the urine always contains glucose
     (c) the arterial PCO_2 tends to fall
     (d) there may be marked hyperlipidaemia
     (e) raised plasma potassium levels indicate an increase in total
          body potassium.

373 Hypoglycaemia is a recognized finding
(a) in normal babies in the first 72 hours
(b) in newborn babies of diabetic mothers
(c) in babies with von Gierke's disease
(d) in babies sensitive to lysine
(e) in babies with galactosaemia.

374 The following forms of xanthomatosis are correctly associated with the usual accompanying biochemical abnormality:
(a) Eruptive xanthomata : raised plasma triglyceride.
(b) Tuberous xanthomata : raised plasma HDL.
(c) Tendinous xanthomata : raised plasma LDL.
(d) Palmar xanthomata : raised plasma chylomicrons.
(e) Premature xanthelasmata : raised plasma LDL.

375 There is evidence for an increased incidence of cardiovascular disease in
(a) familial (monogenic) hypercholesterolaemia
(b) familial dysbetalipoproteinaemia (broad beta disease)
(c) familial endogenous hypertriglyceridaemia
(d) lipoprotein lipase deficiency
(e) familial combined hyperlipidaemia.

376 A raised level of alkaline phosphatase of bony origin is commonly found in
(a) advanced primary hyperparathyroidism
(b) myelomatosis
(c) disseminated malignant disease
(d) Paget's disease of bone
(e) acromegaly.

377 In chronic pancreatic disease
(a) estimation of plasma lipase may be of diagnostic value
(b) the presence of obstructive jaundice is of diagnostic significance
(c) estimation of faecal trypsin is of more value in adults than in children
(d) the islets are spared and diabetes mellitus does not occur
(e) tests involving duodenal intubation are not suitable for routine use.

378 Drugs which have been incriminated as causes of cholestatic jaundice include
(a) aspirin
(b) halothane
(c) chlorpromazine
(d) erythromycin
(e) methyldopa.

379   IgG
 (a) is present in the plasma in higher concentration than all the other immunoglobulins combined
 (b) is the only immunoglobulin able to fix complement
 (c) is the only immunoglobulin which crosses the placental barrier
 (d) does not reach adult concentrations in the plasma until the age of three to five years
 (e) antibodies are usually the first to be synthesized in response to infection.

380   Proteinuria
 (a) of more than 150 mg per day almost always indicates disease
 (b) present only when the patient is standing is never an indication of organic disease
 (c) in which albumin is the predominant protein is probably tubular in origin
 (d) of orthostatic type is associated with a predominant excretion of β-microglobulin
 (e) due to pyelonephritis is usually less than 1g per day.

381   The plasma level of lactate dehydrogenase but *not* that of aspartate or alanine transaminase is typically raised in
 (a) metastatic disease of the liver
 (b) acute leukaemia
 (c) skeletal muscle disease
 (d) pernicious anaemia
 (c) pulmonary embolism.

382   Characteristic biochemical features of Wilson's disease include
 (a) impaired biliary excretion of copper
 (b) raised plasma copper levels
 (c) increased urinary excretion of copper
 (d) deposition of copper in the basal ganglia
 (e) low plasma caeruloplasmin levels.

383   Iron
 (a) is absorbed by an active process in the upper small intestine
 (b) can cross cell membranes only in the ferrous state
 (c) combines with a protein to form ferritin in the intestinal cells
 (d) is absorbed in slightly greater amounts by men than women
 (e) absorption is increased in anaemia even if it is not due to iron deficiency.

Section B

In this section the questions are of the *relationship analysis* type and it is important to read the instructions carefully before attempting them.

Each question consists of two statements linked by the word *'because'*. The first statement is an assertion and the second an alleged reason for that assertion. The correct answer for each is one of the letters (a) to (e) according to the following key:

(a) Assertion and reason are true statements and the reason is a correct explanation of the assertion.
(b) Assertion and reason are true statements but the reason is not a correct explanation of the assertion.
(c) Assertion is true but reason is a false statement.
(d) Assertion is false but reason is a true statement.
(e) Both assertion and reason are false statements.

384 In the SI system it is recommended that plasma total protein concentration be expressed in grams per litre *because* plasma contains a complex mixture of proteins of varying molecular weights.

385 During an osmotic diuresis induced by mannitol the urine leaving the proximal tubule is not isosmotic with plasma *because* its sodium concentration is lower than normal.

386 Inulin clearance is a valid measurement of glomerular filtration rate *because* inulin is not produced in the body.

387 Calculated osmolarity of plasma is normally higher than measured (freezing point) osmolality *because* 100 ml of normal plasma contains only about 94 ml of water.

388 Measurement of osmolality cannot be used to assess osmotic effects across capillary walls *because* proteins contribute negligibly to measured plasma osmolality.

389 Infusion of saline into patients with hyponatraemia and hyper-proteinaemia is not indicated *because* the plasma osmolality may well be normal in this situation.

390 Treatment of diabetic ketoacidosis with glucose and insulin causes hypokalaemia *because* one of the actions of insulin is to cause increased urinary excretion of potassium.

391 In pulmonary oedema the arterial PCO_2 is usually raised *because* exchange of CO_2 across the layer of oedema fluid is greatly reduced.

392   In hypopituitarism the plasma sodium level may be low *because* inadequate secretion of aldosterone causes excessive quantities of sodium to be lost in the urine.

393   Hypercalcaemia does not occur with myeloma *because* the paraproteins do not bind calcium to any significant extent.

394   Jejunal diverticulosis causes folate deficiency *because*, in this condition, the bacterial flora of the intestinal contents is altered.

395   Severe protein malnutrition is a recognized feature of Hartnup disease *because* in this condition there is reduced intestinal absorption and increased renal excretion of several amino acids.

396   In phenylketonuria blood levels of phenylalanine may be normal at birth *because* it does not accumulate in the blood until the baby begins to ingest protein.

397   Plasma iron concentration falls markedly during the menstrual period *because* iron is lost in each period.

398   It has been conclusively demonstrated that symptoms due to iron deficiency can occur in the absence of anaemia *because* cytochrome and other enzymes are among the first to be affected adversely by lack of iron.

399   In affluent countries clinical deficiency of the vitamins of the B complex is rare *because* these vitamins, synthesized by colonic bacteria, are well absorbed from the large intestine.

400   In malignant disease, hypokalaemia is a common accompaniment of hypercalcaemia *because* tumours which secrete parathyroid hormone usually also secrete ACTH.

Answers

Part One

Question	Answer	Question	Answer	Question	Answer
1	(a),(e)	50	(b),(c),(e)	99	(a),(c),(e)
2	(a),(c),(e)	51	(a),(d)	100	(a),(b),(c),(d)
3	(a),(c),(d)	52	(b),(d),(e)	101	(c),(d),(e)
4	(a),(b),(d)	53	(a),(b),(c),(e)	102	(a),(b),(c),(e)
5	(a),(d)	54	(b),(c),(d),(e)	103	(c),(e)
6	(a),(b),(d),(e)	55	(a),(b),(e)	104	(b),(c),(e)
7	(a),(c)	56	(b),(c),(d),(e)	105	(c),(e)
8	(b),(c),(d),(e)	57	(a),(b),(d)	106	(a),(c),(e)
9	(a),(c),(d),(e)	58	(c),(d),(e)	107	(a),(b),(d),(e)
10	(b),(c),(d)	59	(a),(c),(e)	108	(a),(c),(e)
11	(a),(b),(d)	60	(c)	109	(b),(d),(e)
12	(a),(b),(d),(e)	61	(c),(d)	110	(a),(c),(d),(e)
13	(b),(c),(d)	62	(a),(b),(e)	111	(a),(b),(c),(d),(e)
14	(b),(c),(d),(e)	63	(c),(d)	112	(a)
15	(c)	64	(b),(c),(d),(e)	113	(a),(b),(c),(d)
16	(a),(b)	65	(a),(d)	114	(a),(b),(c)
17	(b),(c),(e)	66	(a),(b),(d)	115	(a),(d),(e)
18	(b),(d)	67	(a),(b),(d),(e)	116	(a),(b),(c),(d),(e)
19	(b),(e)	68	(a),(b),(c),(d)	117	All false
20	(b),(c),(d),(e)	69	(b),(c)	118	(c)
21	(a),(b),(c),(e)	70	(b),(e)	119	(a),(b),(d),(e)
22	(b),(c),(d)	71	(a),(c),(d),(e)	120	(b),(c),(d)
23	(a),(c)	72	(a),(c),(d),(e)	121	(a),(c),(d),(e)
24	(a),(b),(c),(e)	73	(a),(c)	122	(a),(d),(e)
25	(b),(c),(d)	74	(b),(c),(d)	123	(a),(b),(d)
26	(a),(c),(e)	75	(a),(d)	124	(a),(c),(d),(e)
27	(a),(b),(d),(e)	76	(b),(c),(d),(e)	125	(a),(b),(d),(e)
28	(a),(c)	77	(a),(c),(d),(e)	126	(a),(c),(d)
29	(b),(c),(d),(e)	78	(a),(b)	127	(a),(c)
30	(a),(b),(c),(d),(e)	79	(a),(c),(d),(e)	128	(a),(b),(c),(d),(e)
31	(a),(c),(d)	80	(b),(c),(e)	129	(a),(b),(e)
32	(a),(b),(c),(d),(e)	81	(a),(b),(c),(e)	130	(a),(e)
33	(b),(c),(d),(e)	82	(c)	131	(c),(d)
34	(c)	83	(a),(c),(d)	132	(b),(d)
35	(a),(b),(d),(e)	84	(b),(e)	133	(a),(b),(c),(d),(e)
36	(a),(c),(d),(e)	85	(b),(c),(d)	134	(b),(c),(e)
37	(b),(d)	86	(b),(c),(d)	135	(a),(c)
38	(b),(d),(e)	87	(a),(b),(c),(e)	136	(b),(c),(d),(e)
39	(c),(d),(e)	88	(a),(b),(e)	137	(a),(c),(d)
40	(b),(c),(d),(e)	89	(b),(c),(d)	138	(a),(b),(d),(e)
41	(b),(c),(e)	90	(a),(b),(d),(e)	139	(a),(c),(d),(e)
42	(a),(e)	91	(b),(c),(d)	140	(a),(c),(d)
43	(b),(d),(e)	92	(a),(c),(e)	141	(a),(d),(e)
44	(a),(d),(e)	93	(a),(c)	142	(a),(c)
45	(c),(e)	94	(c),(e)	143	(b),(c),(d),(e)
46	(a),(b),(d)	95	(a),(b),(d)	144	(a),(c),(e)
47	(a),(b),(d),(e)	96	(b),(c),(d),(e)	145	(a),(b),(c),(d)
48	(c),(d)	97	(a),(b),(c),(d),(e)	146	(b),(c),(d),(e)
49	(a),(b),(e)	98	(a),(c),(d)	147	(a),(c),(d)

Question	Answer	Question	Answer	Question	Answer
148	(a),(b),(d),(e)	198	(b),(d),(e)	248	(b),(c),(e)
149	(a),(c)	199	(b),(c),(d),(e)	249	(a),(b),(e)
150	(a),(c),(d),(e)	200	(a),(b),(c),(d)	250	(a),(d),(e)
151	(b),(c),(d)	201	(a),(d),(e)	251	(a),(b),(c),(e)
152	(a),(b),(c),(d)	202	(b),(c),(e)	252	(b),(c),(d),(e)
153	(a),(b),(d),(e)	203	(c),(d),(e)	253	(d)
154	(b),(c),(d)	204	All false	254	(a),(b),(c),(d)
155	(a),(d)	205	(a),(b),(d)	255	(c),(d),(e)
156	(b),(c),(e)	206	(a),(b),(d),(e)	256	(b),(c),(d)
157	(a),(c),(d)	207	(b),(e)	257	(b),(c),(d),(e)
158	(c),(e)	208	(a),(b),(e)	258	(c)
159	(c),(e)	209	(b),(d),(e)	259	(a),(b),(c),(d)
160	(a),(b),(d),(e)	210	(b),(c),(d)	260	(a),(b),(e)
161	(d)	211	(a),(b),(c),(e)	261	(e)
162	(a),(b),(c),(d)	212	(b)	262	(b)
163	(a),(c),(d)	213	(a),(c),(d),(e)	263	(a),(d),(e)
164	(b),(c)	214	(b),(c),(d)	264	(a),(d),(e)
165	(a),(d)	215	(a),(d),(e)	265	(b),(c),(d),(e)
166	(b),(d),(e)	216	(a),(c),(e)	266	(c),(e)
167	(a),(b),(d)	217	(b),(d),(e)	267	(c)
168	(a),(e)	218	(a),(d)	268	(a)
169	(d)	219	(a),(c),(d)	269	(b),(d)
170	(b),(d)	220	(b),(c),(d)	270	(a),(b)
171	(a),(c),(d),(e)	221	(a),(b)	271	(a),(c)
172	(d),(e)	222	(a),(c),(e)	272	(a),(b),(c),(e)
173	(d),(e)	223	(a),(b),(c),(d)	273	(b),(d),(e)
174	(a),(c),(d),(e)	224	(a),(b),(c),(e)	274	(b),(c)
175	(b),(c),(d)	225	(b),(c)	275	(b),(d)
176	(c),(e)	226	(a),(d),(e)	276	(a),(c),(d),(e)
177	(a),(c),(e)	227	(a),(b)	277	(a),(b)
178	(a),(b),(c),(d)	228	(a),(b),(c),(e)	278	(c),(d),(e)
179	(a),(b),(c)	229	(a),(b),(e)	279	(b),(d),(e)
180	(a),(b),(c)	230	(a),(b),(d),(e)	280	(b),(c),(d)
181	(c),(d),(e)	231	(a),(c),(d)	281	(a),(b),(e)
182	(b),(c),(d)	232	(c),(d)	282	(a),(c)
183	(d)	233	(b),(c),(e)	283	(a),(c),(d),(e)
184	(a),(b),(c),(d),(e)	234	(b),(c),(d)	284	(a),(d),(e)
185	(a),(c),(e)	235	(a),(b),(c)	285	(a),(b),(c),(d),(e)
186	(c),(d)	236	(b),(d),(e)	286	(a),(e)
187	(a),(c),(d),(e)	237	(b),(d)	287	(b),(c),(d),(e)
188	(b),(d),(e)	238	(a),(b),(c),(d)	288	(a),(b),(d)
189	(b)	239	(a),(b),(d),(e)	289	(b),(e)
190	(b),(c),(d)	240	(a),(c),(d),(e)	290	(a),(c),(e)
191	(a),(b),(d),(e)	241	(c),(d)	291	(a),(c),(e)
192	(b),(e)	242	(c)	292	(a),(d),(e)
193	(b),(c),(e)	243	(a),(b),(c),(e)	293	(b),(c),(e)
194	(a),(b),(c)	244	(b),(c),(e)	294	(a),(b),(c),(d),(e)
195	(a),(c),(d),(e)	245	(a),(c),(d)	295	(a),(d),(e)
196	(a),(c),(e)	246	(a),(b),(e)	296	(b),(d),(e)
197	(c),(d),(e)	247	(c),(d),(e)	297	(c)

Question	Answer	Question	Answer	Question	Answer
298	(a),(d)	335	(a),(b),(e)	367	(b),(c),(d)
299	(a),(b),(d),(e)	336	(a),(c),(d)	368	(b),(c),(d),(e)
300	(a)	337	(b),(d)	369	(a),(b),(d)
301	(b),(c),(d),(e)	338	(b),(c),(d)	370	(a),(b),(c)
302	(a),(b),(d),(e)	339	(a),(c),(e)	371	(b),(d)
303	(d),(e)	340	(c),(d),(e)	372	(c),(d)
304	(a),(b),(d).(e)	341	(a),(c),(d),(e)	373	(a),(b),(c),(e)
305	(a),(c),(d),(e)	342	(a),(c),(e)	374	(a),(c),(e)
306	(b),(e)	343	(d)	375	(a),(b),(c),(e)
307	(a),(d),(e)	344	(c),(d)	376	(a),(c),(d)
308	(a),(b),(c),(e)	345	(b),(c),(e)	377	(a),(b),(e)
309	(b),(c),(d),(e)	346	(b),(d),(e)	378	(b),(c),(d),(e)
310	(a),(b),(c),(d)	347	(b)	379	(a),(c),(d)
311	(a),(b),(c),(e)	348	(c),(d)	380	(a),(e)
312	(a),(c),(e)	349	(a),(b),(e)	381	(b),(d)
313	(a),(c),(d)	350	(b)	382	(a),(c),(d),(e)
314	(a),(c)	351	(a),(b),(c),(d),(e)	383	(a),(b),(c),(e)
315	(b),(c),(e)	352	(b),(d),(e)		
316	(a),(c),(e)	353	(b),(e)	**Part Two, Section B**	
317	(a),(b)	354	(a),(b),(d)		
318	(a),(c),(d),(e)	355	(a),(c),(d),(e)	384	(a)
319	(a),(c),(e)	356	(c),(e)	385	(d)
320	(a),(c),(e)	357	(b),(d),(e)	386	(b)
321	(d),(e)	358	(a),(b)	387	(d)
322	(a),(b),(c),(d),(e)	359	(c)	388	(a)
323	(b),(d)	360	(a),(b)	389	(a)
324	(b)	361	All false	390	(c)
325	(b),(c),(d)	362	(a),(b),(d),(e)	391	(e)
326	(a),(c),(d)			392	(b)
327	(a),(b),(d)			393	(d)
328	(b),(c),(e)			394	(d)
329	(a),(d),(e)	**Part Two, Section A**		395	(d)
330	(c),(d),(e)			396	(a)
331	(a),(b),(c),(e)	363	(a),(b),(d),(e)	397	(b)
332	(b),(c),(e)	364	(a),(b),(e)	398	(e)
333	(a),(b),(c),(d)	365	(a),(c),(d),(e)	399	(c)
334	(a),(b)	366	(a),(b),(d)	400	(c)